Drugs of Choice

2020

Selected 2019 Articles from
The Medical Letter on Drugs and Therapeutics®

Published by

The Medical Letter, Inc.
145 Huguenot St.
New Rochelle, New York 10801-7537

800-211-2769
914-235-0500
Fax 914-632-1733
www.medicalletter.org

21st Edition

Contents

Tables

Smoking Cessation

Travelers

Introduction

The Medical Letter, Inc. is a nonprofit organization that publishes critical appraisals of new prescription drugs and comparative reviews of drugs for common diseases in its newsletter, *The Medical Letter on Drugs and Therapeutics*. It is committed to providing objective, practical, and timely information on drugs and treatments of common diseases to help readers make the best decisions for their patients—without the influence of the pharmaceutical industry. The Medical Letter is supported by its readers, and does not receive any commercial support or accept advertising in any of its publications.

Many of our readers know that pharmaceutical companies and their representatives often exaggerate the therapeutic effects and understate the adverse effects of their products, but busy practitioners have neither the time nor the resources to check the accuracy of the manufacturers' claims. Our publication is intended specifically to meet the needs of busy healthcare professionals who want unbiased, reliable, and timely drug information. Our editorial process is designed to ensure that the information we provide represents an unbiased consensus of medical experts.

The editorial process used for *The Medical Letter on Drugs and Therapeutics* relies on a consensus of experts to develop prescribing recommendations. The first draft of an article is prepared by one of our in-house or contributing editors or by an outside expert. This initial draft is edited and sent to our Contributing Editors, to 10-20 other reviewers who have clinical and/or experimental experience with the drug or type of drug or disease under review, to the FDA, and to the first and last authors of all the articles cited in the text. Many critical observations, suggestions, and questions are received from the reviewers and are incorporated into the article during the revision process. Further communication as needed is followed by fact checking and editing to make sure the final appraisal is not only accurate, but also easy to read.

NOTE: The drug costs listed in the tables are based on the pricing information that was available in the month the article was originally published. When the cost of a drug has been updated or added since publication, it is designated as such.

The Medical Letter, Inc. is based in New Rochelle, NY. For more information, go to www.medicalletter.org or call 800-211-2769.

DRUGS FOR
Anxiety Disorders

Original publication date – August 2019

Anxiety disorders (generalized anxiety disorder, panic disorder, social anxiety disorder, and various phobias) are the most common form of psychiatric illness. They can be treated effectively with cognitive behavioral therapy (CBT) and/or pharmacotherapy. Obsessive-compulsive disorder and posttraumatic stress disorder are now considered separate entities in the Diagnostic and Statistical Manual of Mental Disorders (DSM-5); they can also be treated with CBT and many of the same drugs.[1]

PHARMACOTHERAPY

Many different classes of drugs are used for treatment of anxiety disorders.[2]

SSRIs AND SNRIs – A selective serotonin reuptake inhibitor (SSRI) or a serotonin-norepinephrine reuptake inhibitor (SNRI) is generally used for initial treatment of anxiety disorders. These drugs are preferred for patients who also have major depression. Some patients may notice an improvement in anxiety symptoms within 2 weeks, but for others it may take as long as 4-6 weeks. Not all SSRIs and SNRIs are FDA-approved for treatment of all anxiety disorders (see Table 1), but there is no convincing evidence that any one is more effective than any other. SNRIs can cause more adverse effects than SSRIs.

Summary: Drugs for Anxiety Disorders

► A selective serotonin reuptake inhibitor (SSRI) or serotonin-norepinephrine reuptake inhibitor (SNRI) is generally used for initial treatment of anxiety disorders, but it can take up to 6 weeks for patients to notice improvement.
► Benzodiazepines can provide immediate relief of anxiety symptoms, but they can cause dependence and withdrawal symptoms, including seizures.
► Pregabalin appears to be about as effective as an SSRI and an SNRI in clinical trials, with a more rapid onset of action.
► Buspirone has been effective, but it is mainly used as adjunctive treatment.
► Tricyclic antidepressants (TCAs) can be effective, but anticholinergic and other adverse effects have limited their use.
► Second-generation antipsychotics are effective, but they can cause weight gain, metabolic adverse effects, akathisia and, rarely, tardive dyskinesia.
► A single dose of a beta blocker has been effective for prevention of performance anxiety.
► Cognitive behaviorial therapy (CBT) can be at least as effective as short-term pharmacotherapy and produces more durable responses.

Adverse Effects – SSRIs can cause restlessness, sleep disturbances, nausea, diarrhea, headache, fatigue, sexual dysfunction, and weight gain. They can also increase the risk of bleeding by inhibiting serotonin uptake by platelets.[3] QT interval prolongation has been reported with all SSRIs; the risk appears to be greatest with citalopram (*Celexa*, and generics) and escitalopram (*Lexapro*, and generics).[4,5]

Discontinuation symptoms such as nervousness, anxiety, irritability, electric-shock sensations, tearfulness, dizziness, lightheadedness, insomnia, confusion, trouble concentrating, nausea, and vomiting can occur when SSRIs are stopped abruptly; these effects are most common with paroxetine (*Paxil*, and others), possibly because of its potent serotonergic effects, and are least likely to occur with fluoxetine (*Prozac*, and generics) because of its long half-life.

The adverse effects of **SNRIs** are similar to those with SSRIs, but can also include sweating, tachycardia, urinary retention, and a dose-dependent increase in blood pressure. Duloxetine (*Cymbalta*, and others) can cause hepatotoxicity and should not be used in patients with liver disease. Venlafaxine (*Effexor XR*, and others) can prolong the QT interval.[4] Discontinuation symptoms can occur when SNRIs are stopped abruptly, especially with venlafaxine because it has a short half-life.

Both **SSRIs** and **SNRIs** can cause serotonin syndrome, a rare but potentially life-threatening condition characterized by altered mental status, fever, tachycardia, hypertension, agitation, tremor, myoclonus, hyperreflexia, ataxia, incoordination, diaphoresis, shivering, and gastrointestinal symptoms. They can also cause syndrome of inappropriate antidiuretic hormone secretion (SIADH).

Both **SSRIs** and **SNRIs** have been associated with suicidal thoughts in children and young adults, but a causal relationship has not been established, and no increase in suicides has been reported. The consensus of most experts is that these drugs can prevent suicide and are unlikely to cause it.

Drug Interactions – SSRIs/SNRIs and monoamine oxidase (MAO) inhibitors should generally not be used with or within 2 weeks of one another (at least 5 weeks after stopping fluoxetine). SSRIs and SNRIs are metabolized by various CYP isozymes and they interact with many other drugs (see Table 1).

Pregnancy and Lactation – The risk of congenital malformations after use of an **SSRI** during pregnancy appears to be low, and no increase in perinatal mortality has been observed.[6] However, an increased risk of cardiovascular and other malformations has been reported in infants whose mothers took paroxetine in the first trimester.[7] Use of SSRIs in the third trimester has been associated with self-limited neonatal behavioral syndrome, treatment in a neonatal intensive care unit, and a possible increased risk of persistent pulmonary hypertension in the newborn.

The amount of drug excreted in human breast milk is higher with fluoxetine than with most other SSRIs; its long-acting active metabolite is

Table 1. SSRIs and SNRIs for Anxiety Disorders

Drug	Some Formulations
Selective Serotonin Reuptake Inhibitors (SSRIs)	
Escitalopram – generic *Lexapro* (Allergan)	5, 10, 20 mg tabs; 1 mg/mL soln

Fluoxetine – generic
 	
  Prozac (Lilly)
	10, 20, 40 mg caps; 10, 20, 60 mg tabs;
	  20 mg/5 mL soln
	10, 20, 40 mg caps

Paroxetine HCl – generic *Paxil* (Apotex)	10, 20, 30, 40 mg tabs 10, 20 30, 40 mg tabs; 10 mg/5 mL susp
extended-release – generic *Paxil CR*	12.5, 25, 37.5 mg ER tabs
Paroxetine mesylate – *Pexeva* (Sebela)	10, 20, 30, 40 mg tabs

ER = extended-release; GAD = generalized anxiety disorder; soln = solution; susp = suspension
1. Dosage for FDA-approved indications for anxiety disorders. Obsessive-compulsive disorder and post-traumatic stress disorder are now considered separate entities in DSM-5. Dosage adjustments may be needed for renal or hepatic impairment.
2. Inhibitors and inducers of CYP enzymes and P-glycoprotein. Med Lett Drugs Ther 2017 September 18 (epub). Available at: www.medicalletter.org/downloads/CYP_PGP_Tables.pdf. Accessed August 1, 2019.
3. Approximate WAC for 30 days' treatment (caps or tabs) at the lowest usual adult maintenance dosage for GAD. Costs of extended-release paroxetine, fluoxetine, and sertraline are based on the lowest usual maintenance dosage for panic disorder. WAC = wholesaler acquisition cost or manufacturer's published price to wholesalers; WAC represents a published catalogue or list price and may not represent an actual transactional price. Source: AnalySource® Monthly. July 5, 2019. Reprinted with permission by First Databank, Inc. All rights reserved. ©2019. www.fdbhealth.com/policies/drug-pricing-policy.

Usual Adult Maintenance Dosage[1]	Drug Interactions[2]	Cost[3]
GAD: 10 mg PO once/day	▸ Metabolized by CYP2C19[4] and 3A4 ▸ Low potential for interactions; dosage adjustments may be needed with 2C19 inhibitors	$5.40 344.20
Panic disorder[5]: 20-60 mg PO once/day	▸ Metabolized by CYP2D6[4] and 2C9; strong inhibitor of 2D6 and moderate inhibitor of 2C19 ▸ May decrease efficacy of tamoxifen ▸ May increase serum concentrations of 2D6 substrates	20.10 474.60
GAD: 20-50 mg PO once/day **Panic disorder[5]:** 10-60 mg PO once/day **Social anxiety disorder:** 20-60 mg PO once/day	▸ Metabolized by CYP2D6; strong inhibitor of 2D6 ▸ May decrease efficacy of tamoxifen ▸ May increase serum concentrations of 2D6 substrates	8.50 197.60
Panic disorder[5]: 12.5-75 mg PO once/day **Social anxiety disorder:** 12.5-37.5 mg PO once/day	▸ Lower doses of paroxetine may be needed with 2D6 inhibitors	60.00 199.90
GAD: 20-50 mg PO once/day **Panic disorder[5]:** 10-60 mg PO once/day	▸ Metabolized by CYP2D6; strong inhibitor of 2D6 ▸ May decrease efficacy of tamoxifen ▸ May increase serum concentrations of 2D6 substrates ▸ Lower doses of paroxetine may be needed with 2D6 inhibitors	372.80

4. Primary pathway.
5. With or without agoraphobia.

Continued on next page

Table 1. SSRIs and SNRIs for Anxiety Disorders (continued)	
Drug	**Some Formulations**
Selective Serotonin Reuptake Inhibitors (SSRIs) (continued)	
Sertraline – generic *Zoloft* (Pfizer)	25, 50, 100 mg tabs; 20 mg/mL soln
Serotonin-Norepinephrine Reuptake Inhibitors (SNRIs)	

Duloxetine – generic
  Cymbalta (Lilly)
  Drizalma Sprinkle (Sun)
	20, 30, 60 mg delayed-release caps
	
	20, 30, 40, 60 mg delayed-release caps

Venlafaxine –
  extended-release – generic
  Effexor XR (Pfizer)
	37.5, 75, 150 mg ER caps

ER = extended-release; GAD = generalized anxiety disorder; N.A. = cost not yet available; soln = solution	

detectable in the serum of most breastfed infants during the first 2 months after birth. Drug levels of other SSRIs in breast milk are low and are not expected to cause adverse effects in breastfed infants.[8]

Data on the use of **SNRIs** in pregnant women are limited, but increased risks of neonatal behavioral syndrome and perinatal complications have been reported.[9]

Duloxetine is detectable in the serum of breastfed infants. Venlafaxine and its metabolite also can be found in the serum of most breastfed infants.[8]

BENZODIAZEPINES — Benzodiazepines (see Table 2) can provide immediate relief of anxiety symptoms. They are often used as adjuncts

Usual Adult Maintenance Dosage[1]	Drug Interactions[2]	Cost[3]
Panic disorder[5]/Social anxiety disorder. 25-200 mg PO once/day	▸ Metabolized by CYP2C19; moderate inhibitor of 2D6 ▸ Low potential for interactions	$3.60 334.60
GAD: 60-120 mg PO once/day	▸ Metabolized by CYP1A2[4] and 2D6; moderate inhibitor of 2D6 ▸ Avoid strong inhibitors of 1A2 ▸ 2D6 inhibitors can increase duloxetine concentrations ▸ Duloxetine increases concentrations of drugs that are 2D6 substrates	33.00 249.30 N.A.
GAD/Panic disorder[5]: 75-225 mg PO once/day **Social anxiety disorder:** 75 mg PO once/day	▸ Metabolized by CYP2D6[4] and 3A4 ▸ Low potential for interactions; serum concentrations may be increased by 3A4 inhibitors	9.00 443.30

to SSRIs or SNRIs, which can take weeks to become fully effective. Benzodiazepines can counteract the agitation that may occur initially with SSRIs and SNRIs. They are not effective for treatment of depression, which often accompanies anxiety, and many patients find it difficult to discontinue them.

Adverse Effects – Benzodiazepines can cause CNS depression, which can impair cognitive function and driving skills and cause falls in elderly patients. They can also cause dependence and withdrawal symptoms, including seizures, when they are stopped. Benzodiazepines with shorter half-lives (alprazolam [*Xanax*, and others], oxazepam, and lorazepam [*Ativan*, and others]) are more likely to cause withdrawal symptoms. Benzodiazepines are often detected in patients who died from opioid

Table 2. Benzodiazepines FDA-Approved for Anxiety Disorders[1]

Drug	Some Formulations
Alprazolam — generic	0.25, 0.5, 1, 2 mg tabs and ODT; 1 mg/mL soln[4]
Xanax (Pfizer)	0.25, 0.5, 1, 2 mg tabs
extended-release — generic	0.5, 1, 2, 3 mg ER tabs
Xanax XR	
Chlordiazepoxide — generic	5, 10, 25 mg caps
Clonazepam — generic	0.5. 1, 2 mg tabs; 0.125, 0.25, 0.5, 1, 2 mg ODT
Klonopin (Roche)	0.5, 1, 2 mg tabs
Clorazepate — generic	3.75, 7.5, 15 mg tabs
Tranxene T (Recordati Rare)	7.5 mg tabs
Diazepam — generic	2, 5, 10 mg tabs; 5 mg/mL soln[4]
Valium (Roche)	2, 5, 10 mg tabs
Lorazepam — generic	0.5, 1, 2 mg tabs; 2 mg/mL soln[4]
Ativan (Bausch)	0.5, 1, 2 mg tabs
Oxazepam — generic	10, 15, 30 mg caps

ER = extended-release; ODT = orally disintegrating tablets; soln = solution
1. Benzodiazepines should generally be limited to short-term use. Alprazolam is FDA-approved for treatment of anxiety and panic disorder, with or without agoraphobia; the extended-release formulation is only approved for treatment of panic disorder, with or without agoraphobia. Clonazepam is approved for treatment of panic disorder, with or without agoraphobia. Chlordiazepoxide, clorazepate, diazepam, lorazepam, and oxazepam are approved for treatment of anxiety disorder and short-term relief of anxiety symptoms. Chlordiazepoxide (5-10 mg PO tid to qid on the days preceding surgery) and diazepam (10 mg before surgery) are also approved for preoperative anxiety.
2. Dosage adjustments may be needed for renal or hepatic impairment.

overdose[10]; they are generally not recommended for use in patients with a substance abuse disorder. Benzodiazepines are classified as schedule IV controlled substances.

Drug Interactions – All benzodiazepines except lorazepam, oxazepam, and temazepam (*Restoril*, and generics) are metabolized to some extent by CYP3A4. Concurrent use of inhibitors of CYP3A4 can increase benzodiazepine serum concentrations and the risk of toxicity and concurrent use of CYP3A4 inducers can decrease their serum concentrations and possibly their effectiveness.[11] Concurrent use of benzodiazepines and alcohol or other CNS depressants can increase the risk of CNS depression. Concurrent use of an opioid and a benzodiazepine has been

Usual Adult Maintenance Dosage[2]	Cost[3]
0.5-4 mg PO divided tid[5]	$3.60[6]
	384.10[6]
3-6 mg PO once/day	55.60
	601.60
5-25 mg PO tid-qid	48.60
1-4 mg PO divided bid	2.40
	150.80
15-60 mg PO once/day or divided	99.70
	646.80
2-10 mg PO bid-qid	1.80
	204.00
2-6 mg PO divided bid-tid	4.00
	1960.60
10-30 mg PO tid-qid	140.60

3. Approximate WAC for 30 days' treatment (caps or tabs) at the lowest usual adult maintenance dosage. WAC = wholesaler acquisition cost or manufacturer's published price to wholesalers; WAC represents a published catalogue or list price and may not represent an actual transactional price. Source: Analy-Source® Monthly. July 5, 2019. Reprinted with permission by First Databank, Inc. All rights reserved. ©2019. www.fdbhealth.com/policies/drug-pricing-policy.
4. The solution should be mixed in liquid or semisolid food and consumed immediately.
5. Doses up to 10 mg/day may be needed for treatment of panic disorder.
6. Cost for 90 0.25-mg tabs.

associated with a significant increase in the risk of overdose compared to use of an opioid alone.[12]

Pregnancy and Lactation – Use of benzodiazepines early in pregnancy has been associated with an increased risk of spontaneous abortions and fetal malformations.[13,14]

The American College of Obstetricians and Gynecologists (ACOG) considers benzodiazepines moderately safe for use during breast-feeding.[15] Clonazepam (*Klonopin*, and generics) has a long half-life and has caused sedation in breastfed infants. Diazepam (*Valium*, and others) is excreted in human breast milk and with repeated doses, its active metabolite can accumulate in the serum of breastfed infants. Lorazepam and oxazepam have shorter half-lives and are generally preferred for women who are breastfeeding.

PREGABALIN — Pregabalin (*Lyrica*, and others) is approved by the European Medicines Agency (but not by the FDA or Health Canada) for treatment of anxiety and has been widely used for this indication in Europe. Its anxiolytic activity appears to be related to inhibiting release of the excitatory neurotransmitter glutamate from PQ-type voltage-gated calcium channels. In clinical trials, pregabalin has been about as effective as SSRIs and SNRIs in relieving anxiety symptoms, and its onset of action appears to be more rapid, occurring within one week of starting treatment.[16,17]

Adverse Effects – Pregabalin can cause dizziness, somnolence, weight gain, ataxia, dry mouth, blurred vision, and confusion. It is classified as a schedule V controlled substance because of reports of euphoria associated with its use.

Drug Interactions – Pregabalin is not hepatically metabolized and does not induce or inhibit CYP isozymes.

Pregnancy and Lactation – Fetal structural abnormalities and developmental toxicity have been observed in the offspring of animals given high doses of pregabalin.

Pregabalin has been detected in human breast milk; its effects on the breastfed infant and on milk production are unknown.

BUSPIRONE — A 5-HT$_{1a}$ receptor partial agonist, buspirone is FDA-approved as monotherapy for treatment of anxiety, but it is mainly used as an adjunct to other drugs. In controlled trials in patients with generalized anxiety disorder, it has been superior to placebo, as effective as diazepam and sertraline, and less effective than venlafaxine.[18-20]

Adverse Effects – Buspirone can cause dizziness, drowsiness, nausea, and headache.

Drug Interactions – Concurrent use of buspirone and an SSRI or SNRI is common, but the combination could increase the risk of serotonin syndrome. Buspirone is a CYP3A4 substrate; concurrent use of drugs that inhibit CYP3A4 can increase serum concentrations of buspirone and possibly its toxicity and concurrent use of drugs that induce CYP3A4 can decrease its serum concentrations and possibly its effectiveness.[11]

Pregnancy and Lactation – No adverse events on the fetus have been reported in animal reproduction studies with buspirone.

It is not known if buspirone is excreted in breast milk; the manufacturer recommends avoiding breastfeeding while taking the drug.

TRICYCLIC ANTIDEPRESSANTS — The tricyclic antidepressants (TCAs) amitriptyline, doxepin, and imipramine (*Tofranil*, and generics) have been used for treatment of anxiety that has not responded to an SSRI or SNRI. They can be effective, but their use has been limited by anticholinergic and other adverse effects.

Adverse Effects – TCAs commonly cause anticholinergic adverse effects (urinary retention, constipation, dry mouth, blurred vision, memory impairment, confusion), orthostatic hypotension, weight gain, sedation, and sexual dysfunction. They can also cause QT interval prolongation[4] and cardiac conduction delays that can lead to arrhythmias and death when taken in overdose. Cumulative exposure to drugs with strong anticholinergic properties has been associated with dementia.[21]

Drug Interactions – All TCAs are primarily metabolized by CYP2D6; concurrent use of drugs that inhibit CYP2D6 can increase their serum concentrations and possibly their toxicity.[11] Administration of TCAs with

Table 3. Some Other Drugs for Anxiety Disorders

Drug	Some Formulations
Pregabalin[1] — generic Lyrica (Pfizer)	25, 50, 75, 100, 150, 200, 225, 300 mg caps
Buspirone — generic	5, 7.5, 10, 15, 30 mg tabs
Amitriptyline[1] — generic	10, 25, 50, 75, 100, 150 mg tabs
Doxepin — generic	10, 25, 50, 75, 100 mg caps
Imipramine[1] — generic Tofranil (Mallinckrodt)	10, 25, 50 mg tabs
Quetiapine[1] — generic Seroquel (AstraZeneca)	25, 50, 100, 200, 300, 400 mg tabs
extended-release — generic Seroquel XR	50, 150, 200, 300, 400 mg ER tabs
Propranolol[1] — generic	10, 20, 40, 60, 80 mg tabs

ER = extended release; N.A. = generic version was approved on July 22, 2019, but cost is not yet available
1. Not approved by the FDA for treatment of anxiety.
2. Dosage adjustments may be needed for renal or hepatic impairment.
3. Approximate WAC for 30 days' treatment at the lowest usual adult maintenance dosage. WAC = wholesaler acquisition cost or manufacturer's published price to wholesalers; WAC represents a published catalogue or list price and may not represent an actual transactional price. Source: AnalySource® Monthly. July 5, 2019. Reprinted with permission by First Databank, Inc. All rights reserved. ©2019. www.fdbhealth.com/policies/drug-pricing-policy.

other CNS depressants, serotonin modulators, or anticholinergic drugs could result in additive effects. MAO inhibitors can increase the serotonergic effects of TCAs; a drug-free interval of at least two weeks is recommended when switching between a TCA and a MAO inhibitor.

Pregnancy and Lactation – TCA use during pregnancy has been associated with jitteriness and convulsions in newborns.

Most TCAs appear to be safe for use while breastfeeding, but doxepin has been detected in the serum of breastfed infants and may cause sedation.

OTHER DRUGS — MAO Inhibitors, particularly phenelzine (*Nardil*, and generics), have been effective for treatment of social anxiety disorder[22] and panic disorder,[23] but potentially serious interactions with foods and other drugs (including SSRIs) have limited their use.

Usual Adult Maintenance Dosage[2]	Cost[3]
150-600 mg PO divided bid-tid	N.A.
	$514.80
15-60 mg PO divided bid-tid	27.20
50-100 mg PO once/day[4]	16.50
75-150 mg PO once/day	40.70
50-150 mg PO once/day[4]	15.30
	613.20
50-150 mg PO once/day	13.40
	191.50
50-150 mg PO once/day	21.30
	246.40
20-40 mg PO once[5]	0.30[6]

4. Dosage recommended for treatment of depression.
5. Taken about 1 hour before for performance anxiety.
6. Cost of one 20-mg tablet.

Second-generation antipsychotics, particularly extended-release quetiapine (*Seroquel XR*, and generics), have been effective for second- or third-line treatment of anxiety symptoms,[24,25] but they can cause sedation, weight gain, metabolic adverse effects, akathisia and, rarely, tardive dyskinesia.

Although not approved for such use by the FDA, **beta-adrenergic blockers** have been used for many years to prevent performance anxiety such as stage fright. A single dose of propranolol taken about one hour before a performance has been effective in reducing anxiety symptoms without diminishing the quality of the performance.[26] Adverse effects such as dizziness or bradycardia appear to be uncommon with such use.

The first-generation H_1-antihistamine **hydroxyzine** (*Vistaril*, and generics) has been used for short-term treatment of anxiety. It has been effective in some studies,[27] but first-generation H_1-antihistamines can cause anticholinergic adverse effects such as dry mouth, and can also interfere with learning and memory, impair performance on school examinations, decrease work productivity, and increase the risk of on-the-job injuries and car accidents. When these medications are taken at night, adverse effects on wakefulness and psychomotor performance can persist the next day. Cumulative exposure to drugs with strong anticholinergic properties has been associated with dementia.[21]

Gabapentin (*Neurontin*, and others) has been used off-label for treatment of anxiety disorders. No adequate trials evaluating its efficacy for treatment of generalized anxiety disorder are available.[17,28] Gabapentin can cause somnolence, dizziness, ataxia, fatigue, nystagmus, blurred vision, confusion, edema, weight gain, and movement disorders. It is classified as a schedule V controlled substance in some states.

Alcohol is commonly used for self-treatment of anxiety. It is potentially addicting, hepatotoxic, arrhythmogenic, disinhibiting, sedating, and lethal in overdosage, especially in patients who take other sedating drugs such as benzodiazepines and opioids.

Cannabidiol (CBD) products are now widely available in a variety of formulations that are being marketed without FDA approval for various medical conditions, including anxiety (in pets and humans). Their potency, purity, efficacy, and safety are unknown.[29]

COGNITIVE BEHAVIORAL THERAPY

CBT can be at least as effective as pharmacotherapy in adults, and used together they have been more effective than either one alone for treatment of childhood anxiety.[30,31]

CBT can relieve anxiety symptoms in about the same amount of time as an SSRI, but not as rapidly as a benzodiazepine. Even after a relatively short duration of treatment (1-5 months), responses to CBT are more durable than those with a similar duration of pharmacotherapy.

CBT providers may include psychiatrists, psychologists, social workers, physician assistants, nurse practitioners, and psychiatric technicians. State certification and licensing requirements may vary. The National Association of Cognitive-Behavioral Therapists (NACBT) offers four levels of certifications. The NACBT and the Association for Behavioral and Cognitive Therapies (ABCT) both have provider directories on their websites. CBT can be administered in a variety of settings, including individual or group therapy, online (video, mobile application, or texting), or over the telephone.[32]

1. B Bandelow et al. Treatment of anxiety disorders. Dialogues Clin Neurosci 2017; 19:93.
2. A Slee et al. Pharmacological treatments for generalised anxiety disorder: a systematic review and network meta-analysis. Lancet 2019; 393:768.
3. Drugs for depression. Med Lett Drugs Ther 2016; 58:85.
4. RL Woosley and KA Romero. QT drugs list. Available at: www.crediblemeds.org. Accessed August 1, 2019.
5. Citalopram, escitalopram, and the QT interval. Med Lett Drugs Ther 2013; 55:59.
6. O Stephansson et al. Selective serotonin reuptake inhibitors during pregnancy and risk of stillbirth and infant mortality. JAMA 2013; 309:48.
7. A Berard et al. Paroxetine use during pregnancy and perinatal outcomes including types of cardiac malformations in Quebec and France: a short communication. Curr Drug Saf 2012; 7:207.
8. Lactmed. Available at: www.toxnet.nlm.nih.gov/newtoxnet/lactmed.htm. Accessed August 1, 2019.
9. C Bellantuono et al. The safety of serotonin-noradrenaline reuptake inhibitors (SNRIs) in pregnancy and breastfeeding: a comprehensive review. Hum Psychopharmacol 2015; 30:143.
10. CL Mattson et al. Opportunities to prevent overdose deaths involving prescriptions and illicit opioids, 11 states, July 2016-June 2017. MMWR Morb Mortal Wkly Rep 2018; 67:945.
11. Inhibitors and inducers of CYP enzymes and P-glycoprotein. Med Lett Drugs Ther 2017 September 18 (epub). Available at: medicalletter.org/downloads/CYP_PGP_Tables.pdf.
12. I Hernandez et al. Exposure-response association between concurrent opioid and benzodiazepine use and risk of opioid-related overdose in Medicare Part D beneficiaries. JAMA Netw Open 2018; 1:e180919.
13. O Sheehy et al. Association between incident exposure to benzodiazepines in early pregnancy and risk of spontaneous abortion. JAMA Psychiatry May 15, 2019 (epub).

14. SC Tinker et al. Use of benzodiazepine medications during pregnancy and potential risk for birth defects, National Birth Defects Prevention Study, 1997-2011. Birth Defects Res 2019; 111:613.

15. ACOG practice bulletin: clinical management guidelines for obstetrician-gynecologists number 92, April 2008 (replaces practice bulletin number 87, November 2007). Use of psychiatric medications during pregnancy and lactation. Obstet Gynecol 2008; 111:1001.

16. DS Baldwin et al. Pregabalin for the treatment of generalized anxiety disorder: an update. Neuropsychiatr Dis Treat 2013; 9:883.

17. HK Greenblatt and DJ Greenblatt. Gabapentin and pregabalin for the treatment of anxiety disorders. Clin Pharmacol Drug Dev 2018; 7:228.

18. JP Feighner et al. A double-blind comparison of buspirone and diazepam in outpatients with generalized anxiety disorder. J Clin Psychiatry 1982; 43:103.

19. JB Cohn and K Rickels. A pooled, double-blind comparison of the effects of buspirone, diazepam and placebo in women with chronic anxiety. Curr Med Res Opin 1989; 11:304.

20. N Mokhber et al. Randomized, single-blind, trial of sertraline and buspirone for treatment of elderly patients with generalized anxiety disorder. Psychiatry Clin Neurosci 2010; 64:128.

21. CAC Coupland et al. Anticholinergic drug exposure and the risk of dementia: a nested case-control study. JAMA Intern Med 2019 June 24 (epub).

22. C Blanco et al. A placebo-controlled trial of phenelzine, cognitive behavioral group therapy, and their combination for social anxiety disorder. Arch Gen Psychiatry 2010; 67:286.

23. DV Sheehan et al. Current concepts in psychiatry. Panic attacks and phobias. N Engl J Med 1982; 307:156.

24. N Maneeton et al. Quetiapine monotherapy in acute treatment of generalized anxiety disorder: a systematic review and meta-analysis of randomized controlled trials. Drug Des Devel Ther 2016; 10:259.

25. TJ Kreys and SV Phan. A literature review of quetiapine for generalized anxiety disorder. Pharmacotherapy 2015; 35:175.

26. JA Bourgeois. The management of performance anxiety with beta-adrenergic blocking agents. Jefferson Journal of Psychiatry 1991; 9:13.

27. G Guaiana et al. Hydroxyzine for generalised anxiety disorder. Cochrane Database Syst Rev 2010; (12):CD006815.

28. M Markota and RJ Morgan. Treatment of generalized anxiety disorder with gabapentin. Case Rep Psychiatry 2017; 2017; 6045017.

29. FDA Press Announcement. FDA warns company marketing unapproved cannabidiol products with unsubstantiated claims to treat cancer, Alzheimer's disease, opioid withdrawal, pain and pet anxiety. Available at: www.fda.gov/news-events/press-announcements/fda-warns-company-marketing-unapproved-cannabidiol-products-unsubstantiated-claims-treat-cancer. Accessed August 1, 2019.

30. MA Katzman et al. Canadian clinical practice guidelines for the management of anxiety, posttraumatic stress and obsessive-compulsive disorders. BMC Psychiatry 2014; 14 (Suppl 1):S1.

31. JT Walkup et al. Cognitive behavior therapy, sertraline, or a combination in childhood anxiety. N Engl J Med 2008; 359:2753.

32. GA Brenes et al. Telephone-delivered cognitive behavioral therapy and telephone-delivered nondirective support therapy for rural older adults with generalized anxiety disorder: a randomized clinical trial. JAMA Psychiatry 2015; 72:1012.

DRUGS FOR
Atrial Fibrillation

Original publication date – September 2019

Treatment of atrial fibrillation includes anticoagulation, rate control, and rhythm control. US guidelines were recently updated.[1]

ANTICOAGULATION

Anticoagulant therapy reduces the risk of thromboembolic stroke in patients with atrial fibrillation, but it can cause intracranial and other serious bleeding. The decision to use an oral anticoagulant in patients with nonvalvular atrial fibrillation (atrial fibrillation without moderate-to-severe mitral stenosis or a mechanical valve) should be based on the patient's CHA_2DS_2-VASc score. For men with a score of ≥ 2 and women with a score of ≥ 3, treatment with an oral anticoagulant is recommended. Use of an oral anticoagulant can be considered in men with a score of 1 and women with a score of 2, and may be omitted in men with a score of 0 and women with a score of 1. All patients with atrial fibrillation who have moderate-to-severe mitral stenosis or a mechanical valve should be anticoagulated.

CHOICE OF AN ANTICOAGULANT — The non-vitamin K oral anti-coagulants (NOACs; dabigatran, rivaroxaban, apixaban, and edoxaban), also known as direct oral anticoagulants (DOACs), are now recommended over the vitamin K antagonist warfarin (*Coumadin*, and others) in patients with nonvalvular atrial fibrillation. Patients with moderate-to-severe mitral stenosis or a mechanical valve should take warfarin.

Summary: Drugs for Atrial Fibrillation

Anticoagulation

- Oral anticoagulant therapy to reduce the risk of thromboembolic stroke in patients with nonvalvular atrial fibrillation is recommended in men with a CHA$_2$DS$_2$-VASc score ≥2 and women with a score ≥3. It can be considered in men with a score of 1 and women with a score of 2, and may be omitted in men with a score of 0 and women with a score of 1.
- NOACs (non-vitamin K oral anticoagulants) are preferred over warfarin for patients with nonvalvular atrial fibrillation.
- Patients with atrial fibrillation who have a mechanical valve or moderate-to-severe mitral stenosis should take warfarin.

Rate Control

- Ventricular rate control is now widely accepted as an alternative to rhythm control for first-line management of chronic atrial fibrillation.
- Lenient rate control (resting heart rate <110 bpm) appears to be as effective as strict control (resting heart rate <80 bpm).
- A beta blocker is preferred for rate control in patients with coronary artery disease or systolic dysfunction. Verapamil or diltiazem may be preferred over beta blockers in patients with asthma. Amiodarone may be effective when other drugs have failed to control ventricular rate.

Rhythm Control

- Antiarrhythmic drugs, particularly amiodarone, can be used to restore and maintain normal sinus rhythm.
- The treatment of choice for urgent conversion of unstable atrial fibrillation is DC cardioversion.

WARFARIN — Warfarin inhibits the vitamin K-dependent synthesis of clotting factors II, VII, IX, and X.

Dosing – Warfarin requires close monitoring and dosage adjustment to keep the international normalized ratio (INR) between 2 and 3; the INR should generally be measured weekly during treatment initiation and monthly once it is stable. Dosing algorithms based on weight and age are available at www.warfarindosing.org.

Reversibility – Vitamin K (*Mephyton*, and others) can reverse the anticoagulant effect of warfarin.

Table 1. CHA$_2$DS$_2$-VASc Scoring[1]		
Condition		**Points**
C	Congestive heart failure	1
H	Hypertension	1
A	Age ≥75 years	2
D	Diabetes mellitus	1
S	Stroke, TIA, or thromboembolism	2
V	Vascular disease	1
A	Age 65-74 years	1
Sc	Sex category (female)	1

1. In patients with nonvalvular atrial fibrillation, oral anticoagulant therapy is recommended for women with a score ≥3 and men with a score ≥2, unless there is a specific contraindication; it can be considered for men with a score of 1 and women with a score of 2.

Drug Interactions – Maintaining the INR within the desired range can be made more difficult by warfarin's numerous interactions with vitamin K-containing foods (see Table 2) and with other drugs (see Table 3). Warfarin is a substrate of CYP2C9, 2C19, 3A4, and 1A2; inhibitors and inducers of these enzymes can significantly alter its anticoagulant effect.[2] Coadministration of warfarin and amiodarone significantly increases warfarin's anticoagulant effect; the dosage of warfarin should be reduced by one-third to one-half in patients taking both drugs.

NOACs — The direct thrombin inhibitor dabigatran *(Pradaxa)* and the direct factor Xa inhibitors rivaroxaban *(Xarelto)*, apixaban *(Eliquis)*, and edoxaban *(Savaysa)* are all FDA-approved for prevention of stroke and systemic embolism in patients with nonvalvular atrial fibrillation. In clinical trials in patients with atrial fibrillation, all four NOACs were at least as effective as warfarin in preventing stroke or systemic embolism (the primary endpoint) and were associated with lower rates of hemorrhagic stroke or intracranial bleeding.[3-6]

NOACs do not require routine INR-type monitoring or adherence to dietary restrictions. Renal and hepatic function should be evaluated before starting a NOAC and at least annually thereafter. Data on the use of NOACs in severely obese patients (BMI >35 or weight >120 kg) are limited.

Table 2. Vitamin K Content of Select Foods[1]	
Food[2]	Vitamin K Content/Cup
Spinach	889 mcg
Mustard greens	830 mcg
Collards	773 mcg
Beet greens	697 mcg
Dandelion greens	579 mcg
Swiss chard	573 mcg
Turnip greens	529 mcg
Garden cress	518 mcg
Kale	494 mcg
Escarole	318 mcg
Brussels sprouts[3]	300 mcg
Broccoli	220 mcg
Cabbage	163 mcg
Endive[3]	116 mcg
Pickles[3]	75 mcg
Okra	64 mcg
Green beans	60 mcg
Celery	57 mcg
Fennel[3]	55 mcg

1. Adapted from US Department of Agriculture data. Available at: www.ars.usda.gov/nutrientdata. Accessed August 28, 2019.
2. Data for fresh, boiled food. Preparation may affect nutritional content.
3. Data for raw food.

DABIGATRAN — Efficacy – In the RE-LY trial, dabigatran etexilate 150 mg twice daily was superior to warfarin in preventing stroke or systemic embolism (1.11% vs 1.69% per year) with significantly lower rates of both hemorrhagic stroke (0.10% vs 0.38% per year) and ischemic stroke (0.92% vs 1.20% per year). Dabigatran is the only NOAC that has been shown to be superior to warfarin in reducing the risk of ischemic stroke.[7]

Bleeding Risk – There have been multiple reports of spontaneous, severe, sometimes fatal bleeding with dabigatran. In a postmarketing study conducted by the FDA in >134,000 patients ≥65 years old, the risk of intracranial bleeding was lower with dabigatran than

Table 3. Some Drugs That Interact with Warfarin	
Possible Increased Anticoagulant Effect	
Acetaminophen *(Tylenol)*	Fluoxetine *(Prozac)*
Amiodarone *(Cordarone)*	Fluvastatin *(Lescol)*
Capecitabine	Fluvoxamine *(Luvox)*
Cefotetan	Imatinib *(Gleevec)*
Ceftriaxone *(Rocephin)*	Metronidazole *(Flagyl)*
Cimetidine	Phenytoin *(Dilantin)*[1]
Clarithromycin *(Biaxin)*	Rosuvastatin *(Crestor)*
Erythromycin	Sorafenib *(Nexavar)*
Fluconazole *(Diflucan)*	Trimethoprim/sulfamethoxazole
Fluoroquinolones	*(Bactrim)*
Fluorouracil	Voriconazole *(Vfend)*
Possible Decreased Anticoagulant Effect	
Activated charcoal	Enzalutamide *(Xtandi)*
Barbiturates	Nafcillin
Carbamazepine *(Tegretol)*	Phenytoin *(Dilantin)*[1]
Cholestyramine *(Prevalite)*	Rifampin *(Rifadin)*
Colestipol *(Colestid)*	St. John's wort
Dicloxacillin	Sucralfate *(Carafate)*

1. Concurrent use of phenytoin can increase the INR initially, but with long-term use, the INR may be decreased.

with warfarin, but the risk of major GI bleeding was higher with dabigatran.[8,9]

Administration – Dabigatran is primarily cleared renally. Dosage adjustments are recommended in patients with renal impairment (CrCl <30 mL/min, or <50 mL/min in patients concomitantly taking the P-glycoprotein inhibitors dronedarone or ketoconazole).

Drug Interactions – Dabigatran is a substrate of the efflux transporter P-glycoprotein (P-gp). P-gp inducers, such as rifampin, could reduce serum concentrations of dabigatran and possibly its efficacy; coadministration is not recommended. P-gp inhibitors, such as ketoconazole, may increase serum concentrations of dabigatran.[2]

Table 4. Oral Anticoagulants for Atrial Fibrillation

Drug	Usual Dosage	Some Advantages
Vitamin K Antagonist		

Warfarin − generic
  Coumadin (BMS)
  Jantoven
    (Upsher-Smith)
	2-10 mg once/day[2]	Long history of clinical experience
		Once-daily dosing
		Established method for determing extent of anticoagulation
		Vitamin K can reverse anticoagulant effect

Direct Thrombin Inhibitor		

Dabigatran etexilate −
  Pradaxa
    (Boehringer Ingelheim)
	150 mg bid[3]	Lower rates of ischemic or hemorrhagic stroke than warfarin
		Lower rate of intracranial bleeding than warfarin
		Does not require INR monitoring
		Reversal agent available (idarucizumab − *Praxbind*)
		Dialyzable

Direct Factor Xa Inhibitors		
Apixaban − *Eliquis* (BMS)	5 mg bid[4]	Mortality benefit over warfarin Lower rate of stroke compared to warfarin Lower rate of major bleeding than warfarin Does not require INR monitoring Reversal agent available (andexanet alfa − *Andexxa*)

NOACs = non-vitamin K oral anticoagulants

1. Approximate WAC for 30 days' treatment at the lowest usual dosage. WAC = wholesaler acquisition cost or manufacturer's published price to wholesalers; WAC represents a published catalogue or list price and may not represent an actual transactional price. Source: AnalySource® Monthly. August 5, 2019. Reprinted with permission by First Databank, Inc. All rights reserved. ©2019. www.fdbhealth.com/policies/drug-pricing-policy.
2. Initial dosing for warfarin-naive patients should be ≤5 mg once/day. Monitor and maintain INR in therapeutic range (2-3).
3. Dosage is 75 mg bid for patients with CrCl 15-30 mL/min, according to the US label. The American College of Chest Physicians and Health Canada do not recommend use of the drug in patients with a CrCl <30 mL/min. Avoid use with P-glycoprotein (P-gp) inhibitors in patients with CrCl <30 mL/min. In patients taking P-gp inhibitors (e.g., dronedarone, systemic ketoconazole) with CrCl 30-50 mL/min, reduce the dose of dabigatran to 75 mg bid. No dosage adjustment for dabigatran is required with coadministration of the P-gp inhibitors verapamil, amiodarone, quinidine, clarithromycin, or ticagrelor. Avoid use with P-gp inducers.

Some Disadvantages	Cost[1]
Higher incidence of intracranial bleeding compared to NOACs	$6.00
Variability in dosage requirements	64.50
INR monitoring required	10.80
Numerous drug interactions	
Dietary restrictions	
Higher rate of major GI bleeding than warfarin	432.60
Dosed twice daily	
No established method for determining extent of anticoagulation	
Dose adjustment required for renal impairment	
Must be dispensed and stored in original container	
Dosed twice daily	444.20
No established method for determining extent of anticoagulation	
Should not be used in patients with severe hepatic impairment (Child-Pugh C)	
Dose adjustment required for age, weight, and/or renal impairment	
Not dialyzable	

---

4. Dosage is 2.5 mg bid for patients with 2 or more of the following: age ≥80 years, body weight ≤60 kg, or serum creatinine ≥1.5 mg/dL. In patients taking combined P-glycoprotein and strong CYP3A4 inhibitors, reduce the dosage of apixaban by 50% to a minimum of 2.5 mg bid and avoid coadministration in patients already taking 2.5 mg bid.

Continued on next page

Table 4. Oral Anticoagulants for Atrial Fibrillation (continued)		
Drug	**Usual Dosage**	**Some Advantages**
Direct Factor Xa Inhibitors (continued)		
Edoxaban – *Savaysa* (Daiichi Sankyo)	60 mg once/day[5]	Lower rate of composite of stroke, systemic embolism, or CV death than warfarin Lower rate of major bleeding than warfarin Does not require INR monitoring Once-daily dosing
Rivaroxaban – *Xarelto* (Janssen)	20 mg once/day[6]	Lower rates of intracranial and fatal bleeding than warfarin Does not require INR monitoring Once-daily dosing Reversal agent available (andexanet alfa – *Andexxa*)

5. Do not use in patients with CrCl >95 mL/min. Dosage is 30 mg once/day in patients with CrCl 15-50 mL/min. Avoid use with the P-glycoprotein inducer rifampin.

Reversibility – Idarucizumab *(Praxbind)* is FDA-approved to reverse the effect of dabigatran in the event of life-threatening bleeding or an urgent invasive procedure.[10] Dabigatran is dialyzable.

RIVAROXABAN — Efficacy – In the ROCKET-AF trial, once-daily rivaroxaban was noninferior to warfarin in preventing stroke or systemic embolism (2.1% vs 2.4% per year), but did not achieve superiority in the intention-to-treat population.[4,11]

Administration – Rivaroxaban should not be used in patients with moderate or severe hepatic impairment (Child-Pugh B or C). The dose should be adjusted in patients with a CrCl ≤50 mL/min.

Drug Interactions – Rivaroxaban is a substrate of CYP3A4 and P-gp. Drugs that are combined P-gp and strong CYP3A4 inhibitors, such as ketoconazole, may increase serum concentrations of rivaroxaban and

Drugs for Atrial Fibrillation

Some Disadvantages	Cost[1]
No established method for determining extent of anticoagulation No FDA-approved antidote for reversal (andexanet alfa may be effective) Should not be used (less effective) in patients with CrCl >95 mL/min Dose adjustment required for renal impairment Not dialyzable	$363.60
No established method for determining the extent of anticoagulation Should not be used in patients with moderate or severe hepatic impairment (Child-Pugh B or C) Dose adjustment required for renal impairment Not dialyzable	448.00

6. Taken with the evening meal. Dosage is 15 mg once daily for patients with CrCl 15-50 mL/min. Avoid use with combined P-glycoprotein and strong CYP3A inhibitors or inducers.

the risk of bleeding; coadministration should be avoided. Drugs that are combined P-gp and strong CYP3A4 inducers, such as rifampin, phenytoin, phenobarbital, and carbamazepine, can decrease serum concentrations of rivaroxaban and its efficacy; coadministration should also be avoided.[2]

Reversibility – Andexanet alfa (recombinant factor Xa; *Andexxa*) is a genetically modified variant of human factor Xa that is FDA-approved to reverse the effect of rivaroxaban in the event of life-threatening bleeding.[12] Rivaroxaban is highly bound to protein in plasma and is not dialyzable.[13]

APIXABAN — **Efficacy** – In the ARISTOTLE trial, apixaban was superior to warfarin in preventing stroke or systemic embolism (1.27% vs 1.60% per year). Unlike dabigatran and rivaroxaban, apixaban was also superior to warfarin in preventing death from any cause (3.52% vs 3.94%

27

Table 5. Drugs for Rate Control: Dosage and Adverse Effects[1]

Drug	Some Oral Formulations
Beta-Adrenergic Blockers	
Atenolol — generic *Tenormin* (Almatica)	25, 50, 100 mg tabs
Bisoprolol — generic	5, 10 mg tabs

Carvedilol — generic
  Coreg (GSK)
extended-release — generic
  Coreg CR (GSK)
	3.125, 6.25, 12.5, 25 mg tabs
	
	10, 20, 40, 80 mg ER caps

Esmolol — generic *Brevibloc* (Baxter)	N.A.

Metoprolol — generic
  Lopressor (Validus)
extended-release — generic
  Toprol-XL (Aralez)
  Kapspargo Sprinkle (Sun)
	25, 37.5, 50, 75, 100 mg tabs
	50, 100 mg tabs
	25, 50, 100, 200 mg ER tabs
	
	25, 50, 100, 200 mg ER caps[4]

Nadolol — generic *Corgard* (US WorldMeds)	20, 40, 80 mg tabs

Propranolol — generic
extended-release — generic
  Inderal LA (Ani)
  Inderal XL (Ani)
  InnoPran XL (Ani)
	10, 20, 40, 60, 80 mg tabs
	60, 80, 120, 160 mg ER caps
	
	80, 120 mg ER caps

ER = extended-release; N.A. = not applicable
1. Some of the drugs and dosages listed here have not been approved by the FDA for treatment of atrial fibrillation.
2. Dosage adjustments may be needed for hepatic or renal impairment.

Usual Adult Dosage[2]	Some Adverse Effects
PO: 25-100 mg once/day	PO: Cardiac failure, bradycardia, fatigue, ventricular or supraventricular tachycardia, depression, worsening of peripheral arterial insufficiency
PO: 2.5-10 mg once/day	PO: Cardiac failure, bradycardia, fatigue, depression, worsening of peripheral arterial insufficiency
PO: 10-80 mg once/day or 3.125-25 mg bid[3]	PO: Bradycardia, syncope, fatigue, dizziness, orthostatic hypotension, asthenia, hyperglycemia, worsening of peripheral arterial insufficiency
IV: 500 mcg/kg bolus over 1 min, then 50-300 mcg/kg/min; titrate to desired effect	IV: Bradycardia, peripheral ischemia, bronchospasm, injection-site reactions
PO: 25-400 mg once/day or bid[3] IV: 2.5-5 mg over 2 min (up to 3 doses)	PO: Bradycardia, first-degree AV block, fatigue, dizziness, depression, worsening of peripheral arterial insufficiency IV: Same as PO plus injection-site reactions
PO: 10-240 mg once/day	PO: Bradycardia, AV block, drowsiness,depression, worsening of peripheral arterial insufficiency
PO: 10-40 mg tid or qid[3] IV: 1 mg over 1 min (up to 3 doses every 2 min)	PO: Cardiac failure, bradycardia, fatigue, dizziness, bronchospasm, depression, worsening of peripheral arterial insufficiency IV: Same as PO plus injection-site reactions

3. Dosage given as a range; dose and interval will vary depending on formulation used.
4. Capsules can be opened and their contents sprinkled over soft food such as applesauce, pudding, or yogurt and consumed within 60 minutes.

Continued on next page

Table 5. Drugs for Rate Control: Dosage and Adverse Effects[1] (continued)	
Drug	**Some Oral Formulations**
Calcium Channel Blockers	
Diltiazem — generic	30, 60, 90, 120 mg tabs
Cardizem (Bausch)	
extended-release — generic	120, 180, 240, 300 mg ER caps
Cardizem CD (Bausch)	120, 180, 240, 300, 360 mg ER caps
Cardizem LA (Bausch)	120, 180, 240, 300, 360, 420 mg ER tabs
Cartia XT (Teva)	120, 180, 240, 300 mg ER caps
Taztia XT (Teva)	120, 180, 240, 300, 360 mg ER caps
Tiazac (Bausch)	120, 180, 240, 300, 360, 420 mg ER caps
Verapamil — generic	40, 80, 120 mg tabs
Calan (Pfizer)	80, 120 mg tabs
extended-release — generic	100, 200, 300 mg ER caps; 180, 240 mg ER tabs
Calan SR (Pfizer)	120, 180, 240 mg ER tabs
Verelan (Lannett)	120, 180, 240, 360 mg ER caps
Verelan PM (Recro Gainesville)	100, 200, 300 ER caps
Others	
Amiodarone — generic	100, 200, 400 mg tabs
Pacerone (Upsher-Smith)	

ER = extended-release

Usual Adult Dosage[2]	Some Adverse Effects
PO: 120-360 mg once/day or divided tid or qid[3] IV: 0.25 mg/kg bolus over 2 min, then 5-15 mg/hr	PO: AV block, hypotension, heart failure, bradycardia, edema, headache IV: Same as PO plus injection-site reactions
PO: 120-480 mg once/day or divided tid or qid[3] IV: 0.075-0.15 mg/kg bolus over 2 min (max 20 mg), then 0.005 mg/kg/min	PO: AV block, hypotension, cardiac failure, bradycardia, edema, gingival hyperplasia, headache, constipation IV: Same as PO plus injection-site reactions, bronchospasm, depression, seizures, urticaria
PO: 100-200 mg once/day IV: 300 mg over 1 hr, then 10-50 mg/hr over 24 hrs	PO: Arrhythmias (including torsades de pointes), AV block, bradycardia, phospholipidemia, nausea, vomiting, anorexia, fatigue, ataxia, pulmonary toxicity, hepatotoxicity, optic neuritis, corneal microdeposits, skin discoloration, hyper- or hypothyroidism IV: Hypotension, bradycardia, phlebitis at administration site, torsades de pointes (less nausea and vomiting than oral formulations)

Continued on next page

Table 5. Drugs for Rate Control: Dosage and Adverse Effects[1] (continued)	
Drug	**Some Oral Formulations**
Others (continued)	
Digoxin — generic *Digitek* (Mylan) *Digox* (Lannett) *Lanoxin* (Advanz)	0.125, 0.25 mg tabs 0.0625, 0.125, 0.1875, 0.25 mg tabs

per year) and caused significantly less major bleeding (2.13% vs 3.09% per year), but the trials were conducted in somewhat different populations and used slightly different definitions of major bleeding.[5,14]

Administration – Apixaban should not be used in patients with severe hepatic impairment (Child-Pugh C). The dosage should be reduced in patients who have ≥2 of the following: age ≥80 years, body weight ≤60 kg, or serum creatinine ≥1.5 mg/dL.

Reversibility – Andexanet alfa is FDA-approved to reverse the effect of apixaban in the event of life-threatening bleeding.[12] Apixaban is highly bound to protein in plasma and is not significantly dialyzable.[15]

Drug Interactions – Apixaban is a substrate of CYP3A4 and P-gp. In patients taking combined P-gp and strong CYP3A4 inhibitors, such as ketoconazole, the dosage of apixaban should be reduced to 2.5 mg twice daily and coadministration should be avoided if the patient is already taking 2.5 mg twice daily.[9] Drugs that are combined P-gp and strong CYP3A4 inducers, such as rifampin, can decrease serum concentrations of apixaban and its efficacy; coadministration should be avoided.[2]

EDOXABAN — **Efficacy** – In the ENGAGE AF-TIMI 48 trial, edoxaban 60 mg once daily was noninferior to warfarin in preventing stroke

Usual Adult Dosage[2]	Some Adverse Effects
PO: 0.125-0.25 mg once/day IV loading: 0.25 mg (max 1.5 mg in 24 hrs)	PO: Bradycardia, AV block, arrhythmias, anorexia, abdominal pain, abnormal vision IV: Same as PO plus possible extravasation

and systemic embolism (1.57% vs 1.80% per year) and had a significantly lower rate of major bleeding (2.75% vs 3.43% per year).[6]

Administration – Edoxaban is 50% renally excreted and is not recommended for use in patients who have end-stage renal disease or are on dialysis. It should also not be used in patients with atrial fibrillation who have a CrCl >95 mL/min because of an increased risk of ischemic stroke compared to warfarin.[16]

Reversibility – The anticoagulant effect of edoxaban persists for about 24 hours after the last dose. There is no FDA-approved reversal agent for edoxaban, but limited data suggest that andexanet alfa may be effective.[17,18] Edoxaban is not dialyzable.

LEFT ATRIAL APPENDAGEAL OCCLUSION – The left atrial appendage (LAA) is the source of most thromboemboli in patients with atrial fibrillation. In patients undergoing cardiac surgery, occlusion of the LAA can lower the risk of thromboembolism. A percutaneous implant (the *Watchman* device) that closes off the LAA may be considered for nonsurgical patients with atrial fibrillation at increased risk of stroke who have contraindications to long-term anticoagulation.[19]

Device-related thrombus can occur with percutaneous LAA occlusion, usually within the first year after the procedure. A meta-analysis of 66

Table 6. Some Interactions between Amiodarone and Other Cardiovascular Drugs

Interacting Drug	Possible Effect
Amlodipine (*Norvasc*, and others)	Increased serum concentrations of amlodipine
Apixaban (*Eliquis*)	Increased serum concentrations of apixaban
Atorvastatin (*Lipitor*, and generics)	Increased risk of myopathy and rhabdomyolysis
Beta-adrenergic blockers	Increased beta-blocker effect
Cholestyramine (*Prevalite*, and generics)	Decreased serum concentrations of amiodarone
Clonidine (*Catapres*, and generics)	Increased bradycardic effect
Clopidogrel (*Plavix*, and generics)	Decreased conversion of clopidogrel to its active metabolite
Dabigatran (*Pradaxa*)	Increased serum concentrations of dabigatran
Digoxin (*Lanoxin*, and others)	Increased serum concentrations of digoxin
Diltiazem (*Cardizem*, and others)	Increased serum concentrations of amiodarone and/or diltiazem
Felodipine (*Plendil*, and generics)	Increased serum concentrations of felodipine
Ibutilide (*Corvert*, and others)	QT interval prolongation
Isradipine	Increased serum concentrations of isradipine; possible QT interval prolongation
Lovastatin (*Mevacor*, and others)	Increased risk of myopathy and rhabdomyolysis
Nicardipine (*Cardene*, and others)	Increased serum concentrations of nicardipine; possible QT interval prolongation
Nifedipine (*Procardia*, and others)	Increased serum concentrations of nifedipine
Nimodipine	Increased serum concentrations of nimodipine
Nisoldipine (*Sular*, and generics)	Increased serum concentrations of nisoldipine
Rivaroxaban (*Xarelto*)	Increased serum concentrations of rivaroxaban

Continued on next page

Table 6. Some Interactions between Amiodarone and Other Cardiovascular Drugs (continued)

Interacting Drug	Possible Effect
Simvastatin (*Zocor*, and generics)	Increased risk of myopathy and rhabdomyolysis
Verapamil (*Calan*, and others)	Increased serum concentrations of amiodarone and/or verapamil
Warfarin (*Coumadin*, and others)	Increased serum concentrations of warfarin

studies including a total of 10,153 procedures found the incidence of device-related thrombus to be 3.8%.[27]

RATE CONTROL

Ventricular rate control is now widely accepted as an alternative to rhythm control for first-line management of chronic atrial fibrillation. Antiarrhythmic drugs have considerable toxicity, and rhythm control with these drugs has not been shown to be more effective in preventing serious complications than rate control alone.[20] Lenient rate control (resting heart rate <110 bpm), particularly in patients with a structurally normal heart and no heart failure, is easier to achieve and appears to be as effective as strict rate control (resting heart rate <80 bpm).[21] The drugs most commonly used for rate control in atrial fibrillation are listed in Table 5. In some patients, rate control is achieved by AV nodal ablation and permanent ventricular pacing.

BETA-ADRENERGIC BLOCKERS — A beta blocker such as metoprolol or esmolol given intravenously can acutely control the ventricular rate in atrial fibrillation or flutter. Oral beta blockers are often used for long-term rate control. Beta blockers are preferred over calcium channel blockers in patients with coronary artery disease or systolic dysfunction. They should be used cautiously in patients with asthma or decompensated heart failure.

Table 7. Drugs for Rhythm Control: Dosage and Adverse Effects[1,2]	
Drug	**Some Oral Formulations**
Amiodarone — generic *Pacerone* (Upsher-Smith)	100, 200, 400 mg tabs
Dronedarone — *Multaq* (Sanofi)	400 mg tabs
Disopyramide — generic *Norpace* (Pfizer) extended-release — *Norpace CR* (Pfizer)	100, 150 mg caps 150 mg ER caps
Dofetilide — generic *Tikosyn* (Pfizer)	0.125, 0.25, 0.5 mg caps 0.25, 0.5 mg caps
Flecainide[5] — generic	50, 100, 150 mg tabs
Propafenone[5] — generic extended-release — generic *Rythmol SR* (GSK)	150, 225, 300 mg tabs 225, 325, 425 mg ER caps

ER = extended-release
1. For maintenance of sinus rhythm. All of these drugs require monitoring at initiation for proarrhythmias.
2. Some of the drugs and dosages listed here have not been approved by the FDA for treatment of atrial fibrillation.

Usual Adult Dosage[3]	Some Adverse Effects
PO: 400-600 mg daily in divided doses for 2-4 weeks, then 100-200 mg q24h IV: 150 mg over 10 min, then 1 mg/min for 6 hrs, then 0.5 mg/min for 18 hrs; then oral maintenance dosing	PO: Arrhythmias (including torsades de pointes), AV block, bradycardia, phospholipidemia, nausea, vomiting, anorexia, fatigue, ataxia, abdominal pain, pulmonary toxicity, hepatotoxicity, optic neuritis, corneal microdeposits, skin discoloration, hyper- or hypothyroidism IV: Hypotension, bradycardia, phlebitis at administration site, torsades de pointes (less nausea and vomiting than oral formulations)
PO: 400 mg q12h	PO: Hepatotoxicity, possible worsening heart failure with increased mortality, bradycardia, abdominal pain, increased increased serum creatinine, photosensitivity, QT interval prolongation, possible torsades de pointes
PO: 100-400 mg q6-12h[4]	PO: Anticholinergic effects (urinary retention, dry mouth, aggravation of glaucoma, constipation), hypotension, heart failure, ventricular tachyarrhythmias, QT interval prolongation, torsades de pointes, AV block
PO: 0.125-0.5 mg q12h	PO: QT interval prolongation. torsades de pointes, ventricular fibrillation, ventricular tachycardia, bradycardia
PO: 50-200 mg q12h	PO: Bradycardia, AV block, new ventricular fibrillation, sustained ventricular tachycardia, rapid atrial flutter, heart failure, dizziness, blurred vision, neutropenia, QT interval prolongation, torsades de pointes
PO: 150-425 mg q8-12h[4]	PO: Bradycardia, AV block, new ventricular fibrillation, sustained ventricular tachycardia, heart failure, dizziness, metallic taste, bronchospasm, hepatotoxicity

3. Dosage adjustments may be needed for hepatic or renal impairment.
4. Dosage given as a range; dose and interval will vary depending on formulation used.
5. Should be used with a beta blocker, verapamil, or diltiazem for cardioversion. Should not be used in patients with coronary artery disease or significant structural heart disease.

Continued on next page

Table 7. Drugs for Rhythm Control: Dosage and Adverse Effects[1,2] (continued)	
Drug	**Some Oral Formulations**
Sotalol — generic	80, 120, 160, 240 mg tabs
Betapace (Covis)	
Betapace AF (Covis)	80, 120, 160 mg tabs
Sotalol AF (Epic)	80, 120, 160 mg tabs

CALCIUM CHANNEL BLOCKERS — The nondihydropyridine calcium channel blockers diltiazem and verapamil are effective in slowing the ventricular rate in atrial fibrillation or flutter. IV use of these drugs can be complicated by hypotension or bradycardia in patients with underlying heart disease, especially with concurrent use of other cardiodepressant drugs such as beta blockers. Diltiazem and verapamil may be preferred over beta blockers for long-term use in patients with asthma. They should not be used in patients with decompensated heart failure or Wolff-Parkinson-White syndrome.

Unlike diltiazem and verapamil, dihydropyridine calcium channel blockers (all the other calcium channel blockers available in the US) generally have no rate-controlling activity.

AMIODARONE — More often used as a rhythm control agent, IV amiodarone has also been used for ventricular rate control in critically ill patients, and oral amiodarone has been used when other drugs have failed to control heart rate.

DIGOXIN — Generally used only as an adjunctive agent, digoxin can help control ventricular response in atrial fibrillation or flutter, but other drugs are more effective. Digoxin, like verapamil and diltiazem, should not be used in patients with Wolff-Parkinson-White syndrome.

Usual Adult Dosage[3]	Some Adverse Effects
PO: 40-160 mg q12h	PO: AV block, hypotension, dizziness, dyspnea, bronchospasm, bradycardia; higher doses are associated with increased risk of adverse effects including QT interval prolongation and torsades de pointes (can also occur with low doses)

RHYTHM CONTROL

The treatment of choice for urgent conversion of symptomatic unstable atrial fibrillation is DC cardioversion. Antiarrhythmic drugs, particularly amiodarone, are also used to restore and maintain normal sinus rhythm.

ANTIARRYTHMIC DRUGS — The antiarrhythmic drugs most commonly used now to prevent episodes of paroxysmal atrial fibrillation and to maintain sinus rhythm after cardioversion are listed in Table 7.

Amiodarone is the most effective antiarrhythmic drug for maintenance of sinus rhythm, but it has many adverse effects, including GI upset, CNS effects such as fatigue and ataxia, QT interval prolongation, optic neuropathy/neuritis, photosensitivity, and serious, potentially fatal pulmonary toxicity, hepatotoxicity, and exacerbation of arrhythmia. It has a long, variable half-life (usually 40-55 days) and interacts with many other drugs (see Table 6).

Dronedarone, a non-iodinated analog of amiodarone, has been less effective than amiodarone and has been associated with severe adverse effects, including increased mortality in patients with persistent atrial fibrillation.[22]

Propafenone and **flecainide** are generally reserved for patients with structurally normal hearts; they should only be used with a beta blocker, verapamil, or diltiazem. **Sotalol**, a nonselective beta blocker, can prolong the QT interval and can cause torsades de pointes; it should be avoided in patients who have baseline QT interval prolongation or are receiving other drugs that prolong the QT interval.[23] **Disopyramide** is now only rarely used to maintain normal sinus rhythm in patients with vagally-induced atrial fibrillation. **Dofetilide** has been effective in patients with compromised left ventricular function, but it requires in-hospital dose titration and causes torsades de pointes in ~1% of patients[24]; it should not be used in patients with baseline QT interval prolongation or concomitantly with other QT interval-prolonging drugs.[23]

CATHETER ABLATION — Radiofrequency catheter ablation can restore sinus rhythm and may be superior to antiarrhythmic drugs in maintaining sinus rhythm and improving symptoms, exercise capacity, and quality of life. Complications are rare but can be fatal. In symptomatic patients with heart failure and a reduced ejection fraction, catheter ablation may reduce heart failure hospitalizations and mortality.[25]

WEIGHT LOSS

Obesity is a risk factor for atrial fibrillation.[28] In a randomized trial in 150 patients with symptomatic atrial fibrillation and a BMI >27, a structured weight management program decreased the number, severity, and duration of atrial fibrillation episodes compared to lifestyle advice alone.[26]

1. CT January et al. 2019 AHA/ACC/HRS Focused Update of the 2014 AHA/ACC/HRS guideline for the management of patients with atrial fibrillation: a report of the American College of Cardiology/American Heart Association task force on practice guidelines and the Heart Rhythm Society. Circulation 2019; 140:e125.
2. Inhibitors and inducers of CYP enzymes and P-glycoprotein. Med Lett Drugs Ther 2019; March 12 (epub). Available at: medicalletter.org/downloads/CYP_PGP_Tables.pdf.
3. SJ Connolly et al. Dabigatran versus warfarin in patients with atrial fibrillation. N Engl J Med 2009; 361:1139.
4. MR Patel et al. Rivaroxaban versus warfarin in nonvalvular atrial fibrillation. N Engl J Med 2011; 365:883.
5. CB Granger et al. Apixaban versus warfarin in patients with atrial fibrillation. N Engl J Med 2011; 365:981.

6. RP Giugliano et al. Edoxaban versus warfarin in patients with atrial fibrillation. N Engl J Med 2013; 369:2093.

7. Dabigatran etexilate (Pradaxa) – a new oral anticoagulant. Med Lett Drugs Ther 2010; 52:89.

8. MR Southworth et al. Dabigatran and postmarketing reports of bleeding. N Engl J Med 2013; 368:1272.

9. FDA. Pradaxa (dabigatran): drug safety communication – lower risk for stroke and death, but higher risk for GI bleeding compared to warfarin. Available at: www.fda.gov/safety/medwatch/safetyinformation/safetyalertsforhumanmedicalproducts/ucm397179.htm. Accessed August 29, 2019.

10. Idarucizumab (Praxbind) – an antidote for dabigatran. Med Lett Drugs Ther 2015; 57:157.

11. Rivaroxaban (Xarelto) – a new oral anticoagulant. Med Lett Drugs Ther 2011; 53:65.

12. Andexxa – an antidote for apixaban and rivaroxaban. Med Lett Drugs Ther 2018; 60:99.

13. C Dias et al. Pharmacokinetics, pharmacodynamics, and safety of single-dose rivaroxaban in chronic hemodialysis. Am J Nephrol 2016; 43:229.

14. Apixaban (Eliquis) — a new oral anticoagulant for atrial fibrillation. Med Lett Drugs Ther 2013; 55:9.

15. X Wang et al. Pharmacokinetics, pharmacodynamics, and safety of apixaban in subjects with end-stage renal disease on hemodialysis. J Clin Pharmacol 2016; 56:628.

16. Edoxaban (Savaysa) – the fourth new oral anticoagulant. Med Lett Drugs Ther 2015; 57:43.

17. M Crowther et al. A phase 2 randomized, double-blind, placebo-controlled trial demonstrating reversal of edoxaban-induced anticoagulation in healthy subjects by andexanet alfa (PRT064445), a universal antidote for factor Xa (fXa) inhibitors. Blood 2014; 124:4269.

18. SJ Connolly et al. Full study report of andexanet alfa for bleeding associated with factor Xa inhibitors. N Engl J Med 2019; 380:1326.

19. DR Holmes et al. Left atrial appendage closure as an alternative to warfarin for stroke prevention in atrial fibrillation: a patient-level meta-analysis. J Am Coll Cardiol 2015; 65:2614.

20. SM Al-Khatib et al. Rate- and rhythm-control therapies in patients with atrial fibrillation: a systematic review. Ann Intern Med 2014; 160:760.

21. IC Van Gelder et al. Lenient versus strict rate control in patients with atrial fibrillation. N Engl J Med 2010; 362:1363.

22. Safety of dronedarone (Multaq). Med Lett Drugs Ther 2011; 53:103.

23. RL Woosley et al. QT drugs list. Available at: www.crediblemeds.org. Accessed August 29, 2019.

24. JM Abraham et al. Safety of oral dofetilide for rhythm control of atrial fibrillation and atrial flutter. Circ Arrhythm Electrophysiol 2015; 8:772.

25. GA Upadhyay and FJ Alenghat. Catheter ablation for atrial fibrillation in 2019. JAMA 2019; 322:686.

26. HS Abed et al. Effect of weight reduction and cardiometabolic risk factor management on symptom burden and severity in patients with atrial fibrillation: a randomized clinical trial. JAMA 2013; 310:2050.

27. M Alkhouli et al. Incidence and clinical impact of device-related thrombus following percutaneous left atrial appendage occlusion: a meta-analysis. JACC Clin Electrophysiol 2018; 4:1629.
28. YG Kim et al. The impact of body weight and diabetes on new-onset atrial fibrillation: a nationwide population based study. Cardiovasc Diabetol 2019;18:128.

DRUGS FOR
Type 2 Diabetes

Original publication date – November 2019

Diet, exercise, and weight loss can improve glycemic control, but almost all patients with type 2 diabetes eventually require drug therapy. Treating to a glycated hemoglobin (A1C) concentration of <7% can prevent microvascular complications (retinopathy, nephropathy, and neuropathy), but whether it prevents macrovascular complications and death is unclear. An A1C target of <8% may be appropriate for older patients and those with underlying cardiovascular disease (CVD), a history of severe hypoglycemia, diabetes-related complications, a limited life expectancy, or a long duration of disease.[1,2]

METFORMIN — The oral biguanide metformin (*Glucophage*, and others) is generally the drug of choice for initial treatment of type 2 diabetes.[1,2] Its mechanism of action is complex.[3,4] Metformin decreases hepatic glucose production and increases secretion of glucagon-like peptide-1 (GLP-1). It may also reduce intestinal absorption of glucose and (to a lesser extent) increase peripheral glucose uptake. Metformin monotherapy reduces A1C by 1-1.5%, is weight-neutral or causes modest weight loss, and does not cause hypoglycemia.

Cardiovascular Benefits – In a 10-year follow-up of the United Kingdom Prospective Diabetes Study (UKPDS), initial treatment with metformin was associated with a 33% reduction in the risk of myocardial infarction

Summary: Drugs for Type 2 Diabetes
- ► The goal of drug therapy is generally an A1C of <7%.
- ► Oral and non-insulin injectable antihyperglycemic drugs lower A1C by 0.5-1.5%.
- ► Metformin is generally the drug of choice for initial monotherapy.
- ► If metformin alone does not achieve the desired A1C goal, comorbidities or cost may determine the choice of a second drug: a SGLT2 inhibitor or GLP-1 receptor agonist for patients with cardiovascular disease or chronic kidney disease; an SGLT2 inhibitor for patients with heart failure; a sulfonylurea if cost is an issue.
- ► If maximum doses of two drugs are insufficient to achieve glycemic control, insulin or another drug can be added.

and a 27% reduction in the risk of death from any cause, compared to dietary restriction alone.[5]

Renal Impairment – Metformin is contraindicated for use in patients with an eGFR <30 mL/min/1.73 m², and starting the drug in patients with an eGFR of 30-45 mL/min/1.73 m² is not recommended.[6] A retrospective cohort study in 49,478 patients with type 2 diabetes who continued taking metformin or a sulfonylurea after developing renal impairment (eGFR <60 mL/min/1.73 m²) found that metformin monotherapy was associated with a significantly lower risk of major adverse cardiovascular events, compared to sulfonylurea monotherapy.[7]

Other Comorbidities – In a review of 17 observational studies, use of metformin was associated with reduced all-cause mortality in patients with type 2 diabetes and moderate to severe chronic kidney disease (CKD), heart failure (HF), or chronic liver disease.[8]

SGLT2 INHIBITORS — SGLT2 (sodium-glucose co-transporter 2) inhibitors decrease renal glucose reabsorption and increase urinary glucose excretion, reducing fasting and postprandial blood glucose levels. They reduce A1C by 0.5-1%; other beneficial effects include a reduction in systolic blood pressure, weight loss, reduction in cardiovascular death in patients with CVD or high cardiovascular risk, and improved renal outcomes in patients with nephropathy.

Canagliflozin *(Invokana)*[9] – In two randomized, double-blind trials (CANVAS and CANVAS-R) with a median follow-up of 126 weeks in a total of 10,142 patients with type 2 diabetes and high cardiovascular risk, the composite endpoint of cardiovascular death, nonfatal myocardial infarction, or nonfatal stroke was significantly lower with addition of canagliflozin to standard treatment, compared to addition of placebo (26.9 vs 31.5 cases per 1000 patient-years). However, the risk of toe, foot, or leg amputation was higher with canagliflozin (6.3 vs 3.4 cases per 1000 patient-years); this association has not been reported in trials with other SGLT2 inhibitors.[10] Canagliflozin is approved to reduce the risk of major adverse cardiovascular events in adults with type 2 diabetes and established CVD.

A randomized, double-blind trial (CREDENCE) in 4401 patients with type 2 diabetes, albuminuria (urine albumin-to-creatinine ratio [UACR] >300 mg/g), and an eGFR of 30-<90 mL/min/1.73 m^2 was stopped early based on data that the risk of end-stage kidney disease, doubling of serum creatinine levels, or death from renal or cardiovascular causes was reduced by 30% with canagliflozin, compared to placebo. The canagliflozin group also had a reduced risk of cardiovascular death, myocardial infarction, stroke, and hospitalization for HF, and there was no increased risk of amputation compared to placebo in this trial.[11] Based on these results, canagliflozin was approved by the FDA to reduce the risk of end-stage kidney disease (ESKD), doubling of serum creatinine, cardiovascular death, and hospitalization for HF in adults with type 2 diabetes and diabetic nephropathy with albuminuria.

Dapagliflozin *(Farxiga)*[12] – In a randomized, double-blind trial (DECLARE-TIMI 58) in 17,160 patients with type 2 diabetes who had or were at risk for artherosclerotic cardiovascular disease (ASCVD), dapagliflozin did not reduce the composite endpoint of major adverse cardiovascular events (cardiovascular death, myocardial infarction, or ischemic stroke) compared to placebo, but did reduce the rate of hospitalization for HF.[13] In another randomized, double-blind trial (DAPA-HF) in 4744 patients with HF and a left ventricular ejection fraction ≤40%, the composite endpoint of worsening HF or cardiovascular death was significantly lower with addition of dapagliflozin to standard treatment than with addition of placebo (16.3% vs 21.2%), whether or not patients had diabetes.[14] Dapagliflozin is FDA-approved to reduce the risk of hospitalization for HF in adults with type 2 diabetes.

Empagliflozin *(Jardiance)*[15] – In a randomized, double-blind trial (EMPA-REG OUTCOME) in 7020 patients with type 2 diabetes and established CVD, addition of empagliflozin to standard care reduced the rates of cardiovascular death, hospitalization for HF, and death from any cause, compared to addition of placebo.[16] Empagliflozin also reduced the risk of nephropathy (progression to macroalbuminuria, doubling of serum creatinine levels, initiation of renal-replacement therapy).[17,18] In a subset of patients with an eGFR <60 mL/min/1.73 m^2 and/or albuminuria, empagliflozin reduced the risks of cardiovascular death by 29%, all-cause mortality by 24%, and hospitalization for HF by 39%, compared to placebo.[19] Empagliflozin is FDA-approved to reduce the risk of cardiovascular death in adults with type 2 diabetes and established CVD.

Ertugliflozin *(Steglatro)* – There are no completed clinical trials of the effect of ertugliflozin on cardiovascular or renal outcomes.[20]

Class Benefits – In a population-based cohort study (EASEL) in 25,258 patients with type 2 diabetes and established CVD, initiation of an SGLT2 inhibitor was associated with lower rates of all-cause mortality, hospitalization for HF, and major adverse cardiovascular events, compared to initiation of a non-SGLT2 inhibitor.[21] A meta-analysis of 3 cardiovascular outcome trials of SGLT2 inhibitors (empagliflozin, dapagliflozin, and canagliflozin) in 34,322 patients with type 2 diabetes (60% with established ASCVD) found that these drugs reduced the risk of major adverse cardiovascular events (myocardial infarction, stroke, or cardiovascular death) by 11%, but only in those with established ASCVD. Reductions in the risk of cardiovascular death or hospitalization for HF (23%) and in progression of renal disease (45%) occurred independently of the patient's history of ASCVD or HF.[22]

GLP-1 RECEPTOR AGONISTS — Glucagon-like peptide-1 (GLP-1) receptor agonists potentiate glucose-dependent secretion of insulin, suppress glucagon secretion, slow gastric emptying, and promote satiety. They reduce A1C by 1-1.5% and cause weight loss. GLP-1 receptor agonists can reduce the incidence of major adverse cardiovascular events and may have a beneficial effect on proteinuria, but whether they prevent progression of CKD is not clear.

Dulaglutide *(Trulicity)*[23] – Meta-analyses have found no increase or decrease in the risk of major adverse cardiovascular events with use of dulaglutide.[24] However, in a randomized, double-blind trial (REWIND) with a median follow-up of 5.4 years in 9901 patients who had a cardiovascular event or cardiovascular risk factors, the composite endpoint of nonfatal myocardial infarction, nonfatal stroke, or cardiovascular death was significantly lower with addition of dulaglutide to standard treatment, compared to addition of placebo (12.0% vs 13.4%).[25]

Long-term (~5 years) use of dulaglutide has been associated with a reduced incidence of the composite endpoint of new macroalbuminuria, sustained decline in eGFR, or chronic renal replacement therapy.[26]

Exenatide *(Byetta, Bydureon)*[27,28] – In a randomized, double-blind trial (EXSCEL) in 14,752 patients (73% had CVD), the composite endpoint of cardiovascular death, nonfatal myocardial infarction, or nonfatal stroke was 11.4% with addition of once-weekly exenatide to standard treatment and 12.2% with addition of placebo; exenatide was noninferior to placebo in safety but not superior with regard to efficacy.[29]

Liraglutide *(Victoza)* – In a randomized, double-blind trial (ELLIPSE) in children 10-<17 years old with type 2 diabetes, liraglutide (added

Table 1. Advantages and Adverse Effects

Drug Class (A1C Reduction)	Some Advantages
Biguanide (1-1.5%)	
Metformin	Inexpensive; durable A1C lowering; weight-neutral or modest weight loss; no hypoglycemia when used as monotherapy; reduced risk of micro- and macrovascular events
SGLT2 Inhibitors (0.5-1%)	
Canagliflozin, dapagliflozin, empagliflozin, ertugliflozin	Weight loss; reduced systolic blood pressure; no hypoglycemia when used as monotherapy; reduced incidence of CV events, heart failure, and nephropathy
GLP-1 Receptor Agonists (1-1.5%)	
Dulaglutide, exenatide, liraglutide, lixisenatide, semaglutide	Weight loss; no hypoglycemia when used as monotherapy; reduced incidence of CV events and nephropathy; dulaglutide, extended-release exenatide and semaglutide are administered SC once weekly; semaglutide is available in an oral formulation
DPP-4 Inhibitors (0.5-1%)	
Alogliptin, linagliptin, saxagliptin, sitagliptin	Weight-neutral; hypoglycemia rare when used as monotherapy
Sulfonylureas (1-1.5%)	
Glimepiride, glipizide, glyburide	Inexpensive; long-term reduction in micro- and macrovascular complications; reductions in albuminuria
Thiazolidinediones (1-1.5%)	
Pioglitazone, rosiglitazone	Durable A1C lowering; low risk of hypoglycemia

CV = cardiovascular; LDL = low-density lipoprotein
1. Gastrointestinal adverse effects usually decrease over time and can be avoided by starting with a low dose. Use of extended-release formulations may also reduce GI adverse effects.
2. VR Aroda et al. J Clin Endocrinol Metab 2016; 101:1754.
3. Occurs rarely. Metformin should be not be administered for 48 hours after an iodinated contrast imaging procedure in patients with an eGFR <60 mL/min/1.73 m^2 or a history of liver disease, alcoholism, or heart failure, or in those receiving intra-arterial contrast, and eGFR should be re-evaluated before treatment is restarted.

Some Adverse Effects

GI effects (metallic taste, nausea, diarrhea, abdominal pain)[1]; vitamin B12 deficiency[2]; lactic acidosis[3]

Genital mycotic infections; Fournier's gangrene; volume depletion; acute kidney injury; hypotension; ketoacidosis[4]; fractures[5]; increase in LDL-cholesterol; possible increased risk of lower limb amputation, primarily at the level of the toe or metatarsal, with canagliflozin

GI effects (nausea, vomiting, diarrhea)[6]; renal impairment and acute renal failure associated with dehydration caused by GI toxicity; injection-site reactions; possible risk of acute pancreatitis; thyroid C-cell carcinoma has been reported in animals and thyroid C-cell hyperplasia has been reported in humans

Possible risk of acute pancreatitis; fatal hepatic failure; possible worsening heart failure[7]; possible severe and disabling joint pain

Hypoglycemia; weight gain; glyburide has a higher incidence of hypoglycemia and mortality than glimepiride or glipizide[8]

Weight gain; heart failure[9]; macular edema; possible decrease in bone mineral density and increased incidence of fractures, especially in women[10]; hepatic failure; pioglitazone has been associated with an increased risk of bladder cancer

4. PS Hamblin et al. J Clin Endocrinol Metab 2019; 104:3077.
5. D Abrahami et al. Diabetes Care 2019; 42:e150.
6. Slow titration can minimize these effects.
7. M Packer. JACC Heart Fail 2018; 6:445.
8. Because of its adverse effects, many experts no longer recommend use of glyburide (MC Riddle. J Clin Endocrinol Metab 2010; 95:4867).
9. Contraindicated in patients with NYHA class III or IV heart failure.
10. YK Loke et al. CMAJ 2009; 180:32.

Continued on next page

Drugs for Type 2 Diabetes

Table 1. Advantages and Adverse Effects (continued)	
Drug Class (A1C Reduction)	**Some Advantages**
Meglitinides (0.5-1%)	
Nateglinide, repaglinide	Short-acting
Alpha-Glucosidase Inhibitors (0.5-1%)	
Acarbose, miglitol	No hypoglycemia when used as monotherapy[11]
Others (0.5%)	
Pramlintide	Weight loss; reduced postprandial glucose excursions
Colesevelam	No hypoglycemia; decreased LDL cholesterol
Bromocriptine	No hypoglycemia; may reduce risk of cardiovascular events

LDL = low-density lipoprotein
11. If hypoglycemia occurs, it should be treated with oral glucose because these drugs interfere with the breakdown of sucrose.

to metformin, with or without basal insulin) was superior to placebo in reducing A1C over 52 weeks (-0.50% vs +0.80%).[30] Liraglutide is FDA-approved for use in patients ≥10 years old with type 2 diabetes.

In a randomized, double-blind trial (LEADER) with a median follow-up of 3.8 years in 9340 patients with type 2 diabetes at high risk for CVD, addition of liraglutide to standard treatment significantly reduced the composite endpoint of cardiovascular death, nonfatal myocardial infarction, or nonfatal stroke, compared to addition of placebo (13.0% vs 14.9%).[31] Liraglutide is FDA-approved to reduce the risk of major adverse cardiovascular events in adults with type 2 diabetes.

In a prespecified secondary analysis of renal outcomes in the LEADER trial, the composite endpoint of new-onset persistent macroalbuminuria, persistent doubling of the serum creatinine level, end-stage renal disease, or death due to renal disease occurred in 5.7% of patients who received

Some Adverse Effects
Hypoglycemia, especially in patients with severe renal impairment taking nateglinide; weight gain
Abdominal pain, diarrhea, flatulence[6]; transaminase elevations with acarbose
Nausea, vomiting, anorexia; headache; severe hypoglycemia (when given with insulin)
Constipation, nausea, dyspepsia; increased serum triglyceride concentrations
Nausea, vomiting; fatigue; headache; dizziness; somnolence; syncope

liraglutide and in 7.2% of those who received placebo. This difference was primarily due to reductions in new-onset persistent macroalbuminuria with liraglutide.[32]

Lixisenatide *(Adlyxin)*[33] – In a randomized, double-blind trial (ELIXA) in 6068 patients with type 2 diabetes who had a recent acute coronary event, addition of lixisenatide to standard treatment was noninferior, but not superior, to addition of placebo in reducing the rate of major adverse cardiovascular events.[34]

Among 5978 patients with acute coronary syndrome in the ELIXA trial, addition of lixisenatide to standard treatment reduced the UACR by 21% in patients with microalbuminuria and by 39% in those with macroalbuminuria, compared to addition of placebo. Lixisenatide also reduced the risk of new-onset macroalbuminuria, but there were no significant differences in eGFR decline between the two groups at 108 weeks.[35]

Semaglutide *(Ozempic; Rybelsus)*[36,37] – In a randomized, double-blind trial (SUSTAIN-6) in 3297 patients with type 2 diabetes who were at high cardiovascular risk, addition of once-weekly injections of semaglutide to standard treatment was noninferior to addition of placebo in reducing the incidence of cardiovascular death, nonfatal myocardial infarction, or nonfatal stroke (6.6% vs 8.9%). The incidence of new or worsening nephropathy was 3.8% with semaglutide and 6.1% with placebo, a significant difference due primarily to a reduction in persistent macroalbuminuria. Rates of new or worsening nephropathy were lower with semaglutide, but rates of retinopathy complications were higher, mostly in patients with pre-existing retinopathy.[38] In January 2020, the FDA approved use of semaglutide to reduce the risk of major adverse cardiovascular events in adults with type 2 diabetes and established cardiovascular disease.

An oral formulation of semaglutide *(Rybelsus)* was recently approved by the FDA. In clinical trials, addition of oral semaglutide to standard treatment was superior to addition of placebo, the SGLT2 inhibitor empagliflozin, or the DPP-4 inhibitor sitagliptin and noninferior to addition of liraglutide in reducing A1C.[39-45] In a randomized safety trial (PIONEER 6) in 3183 patients at high cardiovascular risk, oral semaglutide was noninferior to placebo in the incidence of major adverse cardiovascular events (3.8% vs 4.8%).[46]

Class Benefits – A meta-analysis of 7 placebo-controlled trials of cardiovascular outcomes with albiglutide (no longer available commercially), exenatide, liraglutide, lixisenatide, and semaglutide found that these GLP-1 receptor agonists significantly reduced the risk of major adverse cardiovascular events (12%), all-cause mortality (12%), and a composite endpoint of adverse renal outcomes (17%).[47] Dulaglutide has also demonstrated cardiovascular benefits.

Pancreatitis – Incretin-based drugs (GLP-1 receptor agonists and DPP-4 inhibitors) have been associated with acute pancreatitis.[48] A review of data by the FDA and the European Medicines Agency did not find a causal link between use of these drugs and pancreatic disease, but both agencies will continue to consider pancreatitis a risk associated with these drugs until more data become available.[49]

DPP-4 INHIBITORS — The dipeptidyl peptidase-4 (DPP-4) inhibitors **alogliptin** *(Nesina)*,[50] **linagliptin** *(Tradjenta)*,[51] **saxagliptin** *(Onglyza)*,[52] and **sitagliptin** *(Januvia)*[53] potentiate glucose-dependent secretion of insulin and suppress glucagon secretion. They reduce A1C by 0.5-1%, are weight-neutral, and are generally well tolerated.

Cardiovascular Safety – DPP-4 inhibitors have not increased or decreased the risk of ischemic cardiovascular events in large randomized trials in patients with type 2 diabetes. In a meta-analysis of 236 trials including 176,310 patients, SGLT2 inhibitors and GLP-1 receptor agonists were associated with significantly lower cardiovascular and all-cause mortality compared to DPP-4 inhibitors or placebo; DPP-4 inhibitors were not associated with lower all-cause mortality compared to controls.[54]

In trials with saxagliptin and alogliptin, more patients were hospitalized for HF in the DPP-4 inhibitor treated group.[55] An increased risk of HF was not detected in either sitagliptin- or linagliptin-dedicated trials.[56-61] In a case-control analysis (CNODES) that included 29,741 patients with type 2 diabetes who were hospitalized for HF, use of incretin-based drugs (DPP-4 inhibitors or GLP-1 receptor agonists) was not associated with an increased risk of hospitalization for HF, compared to use of other oral antihyperglycemic drugs.[62]

Nephropathy – Long-term data on the effects of DPP-4 inhibitors on albuminuria and nephropathy are not available.

Pancreatitis – DPP-4 inhibitors have been associated with acute pancreatitis.[48]

SULFONYLUREAS — Sulfonylureas interact with ATP-sensitive potassium channels in the beta-cell membrane to increase secretion of insulin. The sulfonylureas **glimepiride** *(Amaryl*, and generics), **glipizide**

Drugs for Type 2 Diabetes

Table 2. Formulations, Dosage, and Cost

Drug	Some Formulations
Biguanide	
Metformin[2] – generic	500, 850, 1000 mg tabs
Glucophage (BMS)	
Riomet (Sun)	500 mg/5 mL soln (4, 16 oz)
extended-release – generic	500, 750, 1000 mg ER tabs
Glucophage XR	500, 750 mg ER tabs
Glumetza (Santarus)	500, 1000 mg ER tabs
Riomet ER	500 mg/5 mL ER susp (16 oz)
SGLT2 Inhibitors	
Canagliflozin – Invokana (Janssen)	100, 300 mg tabs
Dapagliflozin – Farxiga (AstraZeneca)	5, 10 mg tabs
Empagliflozin – Jardiance (Boehringer Ingelheim/Lilly)	10, 25 mg tabs
Ertugliflozin – Steglatro (Merck)	5, 15 mg tabs
GLP-1 Receptor Agonists	
Dulaglutide – Trulicity (Lilly)[14]	0.75 mg/0.5 mL, 1.5 mg/0.5 mL single-dose pens
Exenatide – Byetta (AstraZeneca)	250 mcg/mL (1.2, 2.4 mL) prefilled pens
extended-release – Bydureon (AstraZeneca)[14]	2 mg/0.65 mL single-dose pens or powder for injectable suspension[17]
Bydureon BCise[14]	2 mg/0.85 mL single-dose autoinjectors[17]

ER = extended release; soln = solution; susp = suspension; N.A. = cost not available
1. Approximate WAC for 4 weeks or 30 days' treatment with the lowest usual adult dosage. WAC = wholesaler acquisition cost or manufacturer's published price to wholesalers; WAC represents a published catalogue or list price and may not represent an actual transactional price. Source: AnalySource® Monthly. October 5, 2019. Reprinted with permission by First Databank, Inc. All rights reserved. ©2019. www.fdbhealth.com/policies/drug-pricing-policy.
2. Metformin is contraindicated in patients with an eGFR <30 mL/min/1.73 m². Starting metformin therapy in patients with an eGFR of 30-45 mL/min/1.73 m² is not recommended. If the eGFR falls below 45 mL/min/1.73 m² in patients already taking metformin, the benefits and risks of continuing treatment should be assessed.
3. Taken with meals.
4. Cost of one 16-ounce bottle.
5. Taken with the evening meal.
6. Tablets should be swallowed whole not split, crushed, or chewed.
7. Taken with breakfast or first meal of the day.
8. Maximum dose is 100 mg in patients with an eGFR of 30-<60 mL/min/1.73 m². Should not be started in patients with an eGFR <30 mL/min/1.73 m² with albuminuria >300 mg/day or in those with an eGFR <45/mL/min/1.73 m² with albuminuria ≤300 mg/day.

Usual Adult Dosage	Cost[1]
1500-2550 mg/day PO divided bid-tid[3]	$3.60
	100.20
1500-2550 mg/day PO divided bid-tid[3]	665.20[4]
1500-2000 mg PO once/day[5,6]	8.10
	90.60
	4884.30
	N.A
100-300 mg PO once/day[7-9]	494.30
5-10 mg PO once/day[9,10,11]	492.40
10-25 mg PO once/day[9,10,12]	492.90
5-15 mg PO once/day[9,10,13]	281.40
0.75 or 1.5 mg SC once/wk	759.40
5 or 10 mcg SC bid[15,16]	729.60
2 mg SC once/wk[16]	699.80
2 mg SC once/wk[16]	699.80

9. Contraindicated in patients with an eGFR <30 mL/min/1.73 m[2].
10. Taken in the morning, with or without food.
11. Should not be started in patients with an eGFR <45 mL/min/1.73 m[2] or in those with active bladder cancer.
12. Should not be started in patients with an eGFR <45 mL/min/1.73 m[2].
13. Should not be started in patients with an eGFR of 30-<60 mL/min/1.73 m[2].
14. Contraindicated in patients with or who have a family history of medullary thyroid carcinoma and in patients with multiple endocrine neoplasia syndrome type 2.
15. Starting dosage is 5 mcg twice daily, up to an hour before morning and evening meals. After one month, the dosage can be increased to 10 mcg twice daily.
16. The immediate-release formulation is not recommended for patients with a CrCl <30 mL/min and the extended-release products are not recommended for those with an eGFR <45 mL/min/1.73 m[2].
17. Must be reconstituted before administration.

Continued on next page

Table 2. Formulations, Dosage, and Cost (continued)

Drug	Some Formulations
GLP-1 Receptor Agonists (continued)	
Liraglutide – *Victoza* (Novo Nordisk)[14]	6 mg/mL (3 mL) prefilled pens
Lixisenatide – *Adlyxin* (Sanofi)	50 mcg/mL, 100 mcg/mL (3 mL) prefilled pens
Semaglutide – *Ozempic* (Novo Nordisk)[14]	1.34 mg/mL (1.5 mL) prefilled pens
Rybelsus (Novo Nordisk)[14]	3, 7, 14 mg tabs
DPP-4 Inhibitors	
Alogliptin – generic	6.25, 12.5, 25 mg tabs
Nesina (Takeda)	
Linagliptin – *Tradjenta* (Boehringer Ingelheim/Lilly)	5 mg tabs
Saxagliptin – *Onglyza* (AstraZeneca)	2.5, 5 mg tabs
Sitagliptin – *Januvia* (Merck)	25, 50, 100 mg tabs
Sulfonylureas	
Glimepiride – generic	1, 2, 4 mg tabs
Amaryl (Sanofi)	2, 4 mg tabs
Glipizide – generic	5, 10 mg tabs
Glucotrol (Pfizer)	10 mg tabs
extended-release – generic	2.5, 5, 10 mg ER tabs
Glucotrol XL	5, 10 mg ER tabs
Glyburide[26] – generic	1.25, 2.5, 5 mg tabs
micronized tablets – generic	1.5, 3, 6 mg tabs
Glynase Prestab (Pfizer)	
Thiazolidinediones	
Pioglitazone – generic	15, 30, 45 mg tabs
Actos (Takeda)	
Rosiglitazone – *Avandia* (GSK)	2, 4 mg tabs

ER = extended release
18. Starting dosage is 0.6 mg once daily for 7 days, followed by 1.2 mg thereafter.
19. Starting dosage is 10 mcg once daily, up to an hour before the morning meal, for 14 days, followed by 20 mcg thereafter.
20. Starting dosage is 0.25 mg once weekly for 4 weeks.
21. Starting dosage is 3 mg once daily for 30 days. Tablets should be swallowed whole with no more than 4 ounces of water 30 minutes before first food, drink, or other oral drugs.
22. The recommended dosage is 12.5 mg once daily in patients with a CrCl of 30-59 mL/min and 6.25 mg once daily in those with a CrCl <30 mL/min.
23. The recommended dosage is 2.5 mg once daily in patients with an eGFR <45 mL/min/1.73 m^2.

Usual Adult Dosage	Cost[1]
1.2 or 1.8 mg SC once/day[18]	$614.50
20 mcg SC once/day[19]	620.20
0.5 or 1 mg SC once/wk[20]	772.40
7 or 14 PO mg once/day[21]	772.40
25 mg PO once/day[22]	195.00
	385.60
5 mg PO once/day	436.20
2.5-5 mg PO once/day[23]	420.50
100 mg PO once/day[24]	451.20
1-4 mg PO once/day[7]	2.70
	64.60
10-20 mg PO once/day[7] or divided bid[25]	2.40
	90.20
5-20 mg PO once/day[7]	5.10
	49.30
1.25-20 mg PO once/day[7] or divided bid[3]	1.80
0.75-12 mg PO once/day[7] or divided bid[3]	3.80
	26.80
15-45 mg PO once/day[27,28]	4.00
	388.60
4-8 mg PO once/day or divided bid[29]	169.40

24. The recommended dosage is 50 mg once daily in patients with an eGFR of 30-<45 mL/min/1.73 m^2 and 25 mg once daily in those with an eGFR <30 mL/min/1.73 m^2.
25. Doses >15 mg/day should be divided and given before meals of adequate caloric content.
26. Because of its adverse effects, many experts no longer recommend use of glyburide (MC Riddle. J Clin Endocrinol Metab 2010; 95:4867).
27. Should not be started in patients with ALT >3 times upper limit of normal (ULN) with serum total bilirubin >2 times ULN. Contraindicated in patients with NYHA class III or IV heart failure.
28. The starting dosage of pioglitazone is 15 mg once daily in patients with NYHA class I or II heart failure.
29. Should not be started in patients with active liver disease or ALT >2.5 times ULN. Contraindicated in patients with NYHA class III or IV heart failure.

Continued on next page

Table 2. Formulations, Dosage, and Cost (continued)	
Drug	**Some Formulations**
Meglitinides	
Nateglinide – generic	60, 120 mg tabs
Repaglinide – generic	0.5, 1, 2 mg tabs
Alpha-Glucosidase Inhibitors	
Acarbose – generic *Precose* (Bayer)	25, 50, 100 mg tabs
Miglitol – generic *Glyset* (Pfizer)	25, 50, 100 mg tabs
Others	
Bromocriptine[34] – *Cycloset* (Salix)	0.8 mg tabs
Colesevelam – generic *Welchol* (Daiichi Sankyo)	625 mg tabs; 3.75 g packets
Pramlintide – *Symlin* (AstraZeneca)	1000 mcg/mL (1.5, 2.7 mL prefilled pens)
Combination Products	
Metformin/glipizide[2] – generic Metformin/glyburide[2,26] – generic	250/2.5, 500/2.5, 500/5 mg tabs 250/1.25, 500/2.5, 500/5 mg tabs
Metformin/pioglitazone[2] – generic *Actoplus Met* (Takeda)	500/15, 850/15 mg tabs
Metformin/alogliptin[2] – generic *Kazano* (Takeda)	500/12.5, 1000/12.5 mg tabs
Metformin/linagliptin[2] – *Jentadueto* (Boehringer Ingelheim/Lilly) *Jentadueto XR*	500/2.5, 850/2.5, 1000/2.5 mg tabs 1000/2.5, 1000/5 mg ER tabs
Metformin/saxagliptin[2] – *Kombiglyze XR* (BMS)	500/5, 1000/2.5, 1000/5 mg ER tabs
Metformin/sitagliptin[2] – *Janumet* (Merck) *Janumet XR*	500/50, 1000/50 mg tabs 500/50, 1000/50, 1000/100 mg ER tabs

ER = extended release; N.A. = cost not available
30. Doses should be taken 15-30 minutes before meals. Should not be taken if meal is missed.
31. A starting dose of 0.5 mg tid with meals is recommended for patients with a CrCl of 20-40 mL/min.
32. Not recommended for patients with a serum creatinine >2 mg/dL.
33. Not recommended in patients with a CrCl <25 mL/min.
34. Contraindicated in women who are breastfeeding.

Usual Adult Dosage	Cost[1]
60-120 mg PO tid[30]	$41.60
1-4 mg PO tid[30,31]	19.10
50-100 mg PO tid[3,32]	41.60
	90.00
50-100 mg PO tid[3,33]	170.30
	271.80
1.6-4.8 mg PO once/day[35]	251.60
3.75 g PO once/day or divided bid[3]	561.50[36]
	657.00[36]
60-120 mcg SC tid[37]	1093.00
500/2.5 mg PO bid[3]	24.00
500/5 mg PO bid[3]	35.20
500/15 mg PO bid[3,27]	75.00
	N.A.
1000/12.5 mg PO bid[3,13]	195.00
	385.60
500/2.5-1000/2.5 mg PO bid[3]	436.20
1000/5-2000/5 mg PO once/day[3,6,38]	436.20
1000/5-2000/5 mg PO once/day[5,6]	420.50
500/50-1000/50 mg PO bid[3]	225.60
1000/100-2000/100 mg PO once/day[5,6]	225.60

35. Should be taken within 2 hours of waking in the morning.
36. Cost of a 30-day supply of packets.
37. Should be taken immediately before meals that contain ≥30 g of carbohydrate. Insulin dose should be reduced by 50%.
38. Patients who need 2000 mg/day of metformin should take two 1000/2.5 mg tablets once daily.

Continued on next page

Table 2. Formulations, Dosage, and Cost (continued)	
Drug	**Some Formulations**
Combination Products (continued)	
Metformin/canagliflozin[2] – *Invokamet* (Janssen)	500/50, 1000/50, 500/150, 1000/150 mg tabs
Invokamet XR	500/50, 1000/50, 500/150, 1000/150 mg ER tabs
Metformin/dapagliflozin[2] – *Xigduo XR* (AstraZeneca)	1000/2.5, 500/5, 1000/5, 500/10, 1000/10 mg ER tabs
Metformin/empagliflozin[2] – *Synjardy* (Boehringer Ingelheim/Lilly)	500/5, 1000/5, 500/12.5, 1000/12.5 mg tabs
Synjardy XR	1000/5, 1000/10, 1000/12.5, 1000/25 mg ER tabs
Metformin/ertugliflozin[2] – *Segluromet* (Merck)	500/2.5, 500/7.5, 1000/2.5, 1000/7.5 mg tabs
Metformin/dapagliflozin/saxagliptin[2] – *Qternmet XR* (AstraZeneca)	1000/2.5/2.5, 1000/5/2.5, 1000/5/5, 1000/10/5 mg ER tabs
Glimepiride/pioglitazone – generic *Duetact* (Takeda)	2/30, 4/30 mg tabs
Alogliptin/pioglitazone – generic *Oseni* (Takeda)	12.5/15, 12.5/30, 12.5/45, 25/15, 25/30, 25/45 mg tabs
Dapagliflozin/saxagliptin – *Qtern* (AstraZeneca)	5/5, 10/5 mg tabs
Empagliflozin/linagliptin – *Glyxambi* (Boehringer Ingelheim/Lilly)	10/5, 25/5 mg tabs
Ertugliflozin/sitagliptin – *Steglujan* (Merck)	5/100, 15/100 mg tabs
Long-Acting Insulin/GLP-1 Receptor Agonist Combinations	
Insulin degludec/liraglutide[14] – *Xultophy* 100/3.6 (Novo Nordisk)	3 mL prefilled pens[43]
Insulin glargine/lixisenatide – *Soliqua* 100/33 (Sanofi)	3 mL prefilled pens[47]

ER = extended release; N.A. = cost not available
39. Maximum daily dose is 2000/300 mg in patients with an eGFR ≥60 mL/min/1.73 m². Patients with an eGFR of 45-<60 mL/min/1.73 m² should not receive more than 50 mg of canagliflozin bid.
40. Contraindicated in patients with an eGFR <45 mL/min/1.73 m².
41. Reduce the alogliptin dose to 12.5 mg/day in patients with a CrCl of 30-59 mL/min.
42. Starting dosage is 5 mg/5 mg in patients already taking dapagliflozin.
43. Contains 100 units/mL of insulin degludec and 3.6 mg/mL of liraglutide.
44. Should be given at the same time each day with or without food.
45. Basal insulin or a GLP-1 receptor agonist should be discontinued before starting treatment. Starting dosage is 10 units/0.36 mg in patients naive to basal insulin or a GLP-1 receptor agonist and is 16 units/0.58 mg in those on basal insulin or a GLP-1 receptor agonist; titrate up or down by 2 units every 3-4 days to achieve desired fasting plasma glucose.

Usual Adult Dosage	Cost[1]
500/50-500/150 mg PO bid[3,39]	$494.30
1000/100-1000/300 mg PO once/day[6,7,39]	494.30
500/5-1000/10 mg PO once/day[6,7,11,38]	492.40
500/5-1000/12.5 mg PO bid[3,40]	492.90
1000/5-1000/25 mg PO once/day[6,7,40]	246.40
500/2.5-1000/7.5 mg PO bid[3,13]	281.40
1000/5/5-2000/10/5 mg PO once/day[6,7,11]	N.A.
2/30-4/30 mg PO once/day[7,27]	390.50 593.80
25/15-25/45 mg PO once/day[10,27,28,41]	195.00 385.60
10/5 mg PO once/day[10,11,42]	492.40
10/5-25/5 mg PO once/day[10,12]	539.30
5/100-15/100 mg PO once/day[10,13]	549.90
16-50 units SC once/day[44,45]	831.90[46]
15-60 units SC once/day[48,49]	565.40[46]

46. Cost of 30 days' treatment for a patient using *Xultophy* 40 units/1.44 mg daily or *Soliqua* 40 units/ 13.3 mcg daily.
47. Contains 100 units/mL of insulin glargine and 33 mcg/mL of lixisenatide.
48. Within one hour before first meal of the day.
49. Basal insulin or a GLP-1 receptor agonist should be discontinued before starting treatment. Starting dosage is 15 units/5 mcg in patients naive to basal insulin or a GLP-1 receptor agonist, on <30 units of basal insulin, or on a GLP-1 receptor agonist, and is 30 units/10 mcg in those on 30-60 units of basal insulin; titrate up or down by 2-4 units/week to achieve desired fasting plasma glucose.

(*Glucotrol*, and others), and **glyburide** (*Glynase Prestab*, and others), reduce A1C by 1-1.5%, but the reductions are less durable than those with metformin, and these drugs can cause weight gain and hypoglycemia. A meta-analysis of long-term trials found that use of sulfonylureas was associated with a reduced risk of microvascular and macrovascular complications of diabetes.[63] Their effectiveness and low cost have led to wide use of these drugs as second-line agents.

Cardiovascular Safety – Until recently, the cardiovascular safety of sulfonylureas was suspect because of a 1970 report,[64] but in a recent randomized controlled trial (CAROLINA) in 6042 patients with type 2 diabetes and increased cardiovascular risk, addition of glimepiride to standard treatment was noninferior to addition of the DPP-4 inhibitor linagliptin in cardiovascular safety.[65] In an earlier trial (CARMELINA), addition of linagliptin to standard treatment was noninferior to addition of placebo in cardiovascular safety.[66]

THIAZOLIDINEDIONES (TZDs) — Pioglitazone (*Actos*, and generics) and **rosiglitazone** *(Avandia)* increase the insulin sensitivity of adipose tissue, skeletal muscle, and the liver, and reduce hepatic glucose production. They reduce A1C by 1-1.5%. Whether the benefits of TZDs outweigh their risks (weight gain, heart failure, anemia, increased fracture risk) remains unclear.

Cardiovascular Risk – Both pioglitazone and rosiglitazone have been associated with an increased risk of heart failure,[67] but in a randomized controlled trial, there was no significant difference between rosiglitazone and metformin plus a sulfonylurea in the risk of cardiovascular death, myocardial infarction, or stroke.[68] Restrictions placed on rosiglitazone in 2010 because of concerns about its cardiovascular safety have been lifted.[69]

MEGLITINIDES — Nateglinide and **repaglinide**, although structurally different from the sulfonylureas, also bind to ATP-sensitive potassium channels on beta cells and increase insulin release.

Repaglinide is more effective than nateglinide in lowering A1C (1% vs 0.5%) and has the advantage of being safe for use in patients with renal failure. Both are rapidly absorbed and cleared; plasma levels of insulin peak 30-60 minutes after each dose and multiple daily doses are required. These drugs permit more dosing flexibility than sulfonylureas, but they also can cause hypoglycemia and they have not been shown to reduce microvascular complications or to have a beneficial effect on cardiovascular outcomes.

ALPHA-GLUCOSIDASE INHIBITORS — **Acarbose** (*Precose*, and generics) and **miglitol** (*Glyset*, and generics) inhibit the alpha-glucosidase enzymes that line the brush border of the small intestine, interfering with hydrolysis of carbohydrates and delaying absorption of glucose and other monosaccharides. They reduce A1C by 0.5-1%. To lower postprandial glucose concentrations, these drugs must be taken with each meal.

OTHER AGENTS — Other FDA-approved agents for type 2 diabetes include the immediate-release formulation of the ergot-derived dopamine agonist **bromocriptine** mesylate *(Cycloset)*, the bile acid sequestrant **colesevelam**[70] (*Welchol*, and generics) and the subcutaneously-injected amylin mimetic **pramlintide** *(Symlin)*. None of these agents are recommended as monotherapy and they are minimally effective at reducing A1C (~0.5% reduction).

INSULIN — Many patients with type 2 diabetes eventually require insulin to achieve glycemic control. Insulin therapy for type 2 diabetes was reviewed in a previous issue.[71]

PREGNANCY — Insulin is the drug of choice for treatment of pregnant women with type 2 diabetes because it does not cross the placenta. It is excreted in human breast milk, but women who use insulin can breastfeed safely. Metformin also appears to be relatively safe for use in pregnant women.[72] Data on the safety of other antihyperglycemic drugs during pregnancy are insufficient to recommend their use.

Drugs for Type 2 Diabetes

1. American Diabetes Association. Professional practice committee for the standards of medical care in diabetes – 2019. Diabetes Care 2019; 42:(Suppl 1).
2. AJ Garber et al. Consensus statement by the American Association of Clinical Endocrinologists and American College of Endocrinology on the comprehensive type 2 diabetes management algorithm – 2019 executive summary. Endocr Pract 2019; 25:69.
3. E Ferrannini. The target of metformin in type 2 diabetes. N Engl J Med 2014; 371:1547.
4. JB Buse et al. The primary glucose-lowering effect of metformin resides in the gut, not the circulation: results from short-term pharmacokinetic and 12-week dose-ranging studies. Diabetes Care 2016; 39:198.
5. RR Holman et al. 10-year follow-up of intensive glucose control in type 2 diabetes. N Engl J Med 2008; 359:1577.
6. FDA Drug Safety Communication: FDA revises warnings regarding use of the diabetes medicine metformin in certain patients with reduced kidney function. Available at: www.fda.gov/drugs/drugsafety/ucm493244.htm. Accessed October 23, 2019.
7. CL Roumie et al. Association of treatment with metformin vs sulfonylurea with major adverse cardiovascular events among patients with diabetes and reduced kidney function. JAMA 2019; 322:1167.
8. MJ Crowley et al. Clinical outcomes of metformin use in populations with chronic kidney disease, congestive heart failure, or chronic liver disease: a systematic review. Ann Intern Med 2017; 166:191.
9. Canagliflozin (Invokana) for type 2 diabetes. Med Lett Drugs Ther 2013; 55:37.
10. B Neal et al. Canagliflozin and cardiovascular and renal events in type 2 diabetes. N Engl J Med 2017; 377:644.
11. V Perkovic et al. Canagliflozin and renal outcomes in type 2 diabetes and nephropathy. N Engl J Med 2019; 380;2295.
12. Dapagliflozin (Farxiga) for type 2 diabetes. Med Lett Drugs Ther 2014; 56:13.
13. SD Wiviott et al. Dapagliflozin and cardiovascular outcomes in type 2 diabetes. N Engl J Med 2019; 380:347.
14. JJV McMurray et al. Dapagliflozin in patients with heart failure and reduced ejection fraction. N Engl J Med. Sept 2019 (epub).
15. Empagliflozin (Jardiance) for diabetes. Med Lett Drugs Ther 2014; 56:99.
16. B Zinman et al. Empagliflozin, cardiovascular outcomes, and mortality in type 2 diabetes. N Engl J Med 2015; 373:2117.
17. C Wanner et al. Empagliflozin and progression of kidney disease in type 2 diabetes. N Engl J Med 2016; 375:323.
18. SGLT2 inhibitors and renal function. Med Lett Drugs Ther 2016; 58:91.
19. C Wanner et al. Empagliflozin and clinical outcomes in patients with type 2 diabetes mellitus, established cardiovascular disease, and chronic kidney disease. Circulation 2018; 137:119.
20. Ertugliflozin for type 2 diabetes. Med Lett Drugs Ther 2018; 60:70.
21. JA Udell et al. Cardiovascular outcomes and risks after initiation of a sodium glucose cotransporter 2 inhibitor: results from the EASEL population-based cohort study (evidence for cardiovascular outcomes with sodium glucose cotransporter 2 inhibitors in the real world). Circulation 2018; 137:1450.

22. TA Zelniker et al. SGLT2 inhibitors for primary and secondary prevention of cardiovascular and renal outcomes in type 2 diabetes: a systematic review and meta-analysis of cardiovascular outcome trials. Lancet 2019; 393:31.
23. Two new GLP-1 receptor agonists for diabetes. Med Lett Drugs Ther 2014; 56:109.
24. KC Ferdinand et al. Cardiovascular safety for once-weekly dulaglutide in type 2 diabetes: a pre-specified meta-analysis of prospectively adjudicated cardiovascular events. Cardiovasc Diabetol 2016; 15:38.
25. HC Gerstein et al. Dulaglutide and cardiovascular outcomes in type 2 diabetes (REWIND): a double-blind, randomised placebo-controlled trial. Lancet 2019; 394:121.
26. HC Gerstein et al. Dulaglutide and renal outcomes in type 2 diabetes: an exploratory analysis of the REWIND randomised, placebo-controlled trial. Lancet 2019; 394:131.
27. Exenatide (Byetta) for type 2 diabetes. Med Lett Drugs Ther 2005; 47:45.
28. Extended-release exenatide (Bydureon) for type 2 diabetes. Med Lett Drugs Ther 2012; 54:21.
29. RR Holman et al. Effects of once-weekly exenatide on cardiovascular outcomes in type 2 diabetes. N Engl J Med 2017; 377:1228.
30. WV Tamborlane et al. Liraglutide in children and adolescents with type 2 diabetes. N Engl J Med 2019; 381:637.
31. SP Marso et al. Liraglutide and cardiovascular outcomes in type 2 diabetes. N Engl J Med 2016; 375:311.
32. JFE Mann et al. Liraglutide and renal outcomes in type 2 diabetes. N Engl J Med 2017; 377:839.
33. Lixisenatide for type 2 diabetes. Med Lett Drugs Ther 2017; 59:19.
34. MA Pfeffer et al. Lixisenatide in patients with type 2 diabetes and acute coronary syndrome. N Engl J Med 2015; 373:2247.
35. MHA Muskiet et al. Lixisenatide and renal outcomes in patients with type 2 diabetes and acute coronary syndrome: an exploratory analysis of the ELIXA randomised, placebo-controlled trial. Lancet Diabetes Endocrinol 2018; 6:859.
36. Semaglutide (Ozempic) - another injectable GLP-1 receptor agonist for type 2 diabetes. Med Lett Drugs Ther 2018; 60:19.
37. Oral semaglutide (Rybelsus) for type 2 diabetes. Med Lett Drugs Ther 2019; 61:166.
38. SP Marso et al. Semaglutide and cardiovascular outcomes in patients with type 2 diabetes. N Engl J Med 2016; 375:1834.
39. R Pratley et al. Oral semaglutide versus subcutaneous liraglutide and placebo in type 2 diabetes (PIONEER 4): a randomised, double-blind, phase 3a trial. Lancet 2019; 394:39.
40. VR Aroda et al. PIONEER 1: randomized clinical trial of the efficacy and safety of oral semaglutide monotherapy in comparison with placebo in patients with type 2 diabetes. Diabetes Care 2019; 42:1724.
41. HW Rodbard et al. Oral semaglutide versus empagliflozin in patients with type 2 diabetes uncontrolled on metformin: the PIONEER 2 trial. Diabetes Care 2019 Sep 17 (epub).
42. J Rosenstock et al. Effect of additional oral semaglutide vs sitagliptin on glycated hemoglobin in adults with type 2 diabetes uncontrolled with metformin alone or with sulfonylurea: the PIONEER 3 randomized clinical trial. JAMA 2019; 321:1466.

43. O Mosenzon et al. Efficacy and safety of oral semaglutide in patients with type 2 diabetes and moderate renal impairment (PIONEER 5): a placebo-controlled, randomised, phase 3a trial. Lancet Diabetes Endocrinol 2019; 7:515.
44. TR Pieber et al. Efficacy and safety of oral semaglutide with flexible dose adjustment versus sitagliptin in type 2 diabetes (PIONEER 7): a multicentre, open-label, randomised, phase 3a trial. Lancet Diabetes Endocrinol 2019; 7:528.
45. B Zinman et al. Efficacy, safety, and tolerability of oral semaglutide versus placebo added to insulin with or without metformin in patients with type 2 diabetes: the PIONEER 8 Trial. Diabetes Care 2019 Sep 17 (epub).
46. M Husain et al. Oral semaglutide and cardiovascular outcomes in patients with type 2 diabetes. N Engl J Med. 2019; 381:841.
47. SL Kristensen et al. Cardiovascular, mortality, and kidney outcomes with GLP-1 receptor agonists in patients with type 2 diabetes: a systematic review and meta-analysis of cardiovascular outcome trials. Lancet Diabetes Endocrinol 2019; 7:776.
48. PC Butler et al. A critical analysis of the clinical use of incretin-based therapies: are the GLP-1 therapies safe? Diabetes Care 2013; 36:2118.
49. AG Egan et al. Pancreatic safety of incretin-based drugs–FDA and EMA assessment. N Engl J Med 2014; 370:794.
50. Alogliptin (Nesina) for type 2 diabetes. Med Lett Drugs Ther 2013; 55:41.
51. Linagliptin (Tradjenta) – a new DPP-4 inhibitor for type 2 diabetes. Med Lett Drugs Ther 2011; 53:49.
52. Saxagliptin (Onglyza) for type 2 diabetes. Med Lett Drugs Ther 2009; 51:85.
53. Sitagliptin (Januvia) for type 2 diabetes. Med Lett Drugs Ther 2007; 49:1.
54. SL Zheng et al. Association between use of sodium-glucose cotransporter 2 inhibitors, glucagon-like peptide 1 agonists, and dipeptidyl peptidase 4 inhibitors with all-cause mortality in patients with type 2 diabetes: a systematic review and meta-analysis. JAMA 2018; 319:1580.
55. FDA Drug Safety Communication: FDA adds warnings about heart failure risk to labels of type 2 diabetes medicines containing saxagliptin and alogliptin. Available at: www.fda.gov/drugs/drug-safety-and-availability/fda-drug-safety-communication-fda-adds-warnings-about-heart-failure-risk-labels-type-2-diabetes. Accessed October 24, 2019.
56. BM Scirica et al. Saxagliptin and cardiovascular outcomes in patients with type 2 diabetes mellitus. N Engl J Med 2013; 369:1317.
57. WB White et al. Alogliptin after acute coronary syndrome in patients with type 2 diabetes. N Engl J Med 2013; 369:1327.
58. JB Green et al. Effect of sitagliptin on cardiovascular outcomes in type 2 diabetes. N Engl J Med 2015; 373:232.
59. DK McGuire et al. Linagliptin effects on heart failure and related outcomes in individuals with type 2 diabetes mellitus at high cardiovascular and renal risk in CARMELINA. Circulation 2018; 139:351.
60. VP Sanon et al. Play of chance versus concerns regarding dipeptidyl peptidase-4 inhibitors: heart failure and diabetes. Clin Diabetes 2014; 32:121.
61. KB Filion and S Suissa. DPP-4 inhibitors and heart failure: some reassurance, some uncertainty. Diabetes Care 2016; 39:735.

62. KB Filion et al. A multicenter observational study of incretin-based drugs and heart failure. N Engl J Med 2016: 374:1145.

63. D Varvaki Rados et al. The association between sulfonylurea use and all-cause and cardiovascular mortality: a meta-analysis with trial sequential analysis of randomized clinical trials. PLoS Med 2016; 13:e1001992.

64. DJ Wexler. Sulfonylureas and cardiovascular safety: the final verdict. JAMA 2019; 322:1147.

65. J Rosenstock et al. Effect of linagliptin vs glimepiride on major adverse cardiovascular outcomes in patients with type 2 diabetes: the CAROLINA randomized clinical trial. JAMA 2019; 322:1155.

66. J Rosenstock et al. Effect of linagliptin vs placebo on major cardiovascular outcomes in adults with type 2 diabetes and high cardiovascular and renal risk: the CARMELINA randomized clinical trial. JAMA 2019; 321:69.

67. AV Hernandez et al. Thiazolidinediones and risk of heart failure in patients with or at high risk of type 2 diabetes mellitus: a meta-analysis and meta-regression analysis of placebo-controlled randomized clinical trials. Am J Cardiovasc Drugs 2011; 11:115.

68. KW Mahaffey et al. Results of a reevaluation of cardiovascular outcomes in the RECORD trial. Am Heart J 2013; 166:240.

69. In brief: Rosiglitazone (Avandia) unbound. Med Lett Drugs Ther 2014; 56:12.

70. In brief: a new indication for colesevelam (Welchol). Med Lett Drugs Ther 2008; 50:33.

71. Insulins for type 2 diabetes. Med Lett Drugs Ther 2019; 61:65.

72. KC Bishop et al. Pharmacologic treatment of diabetes in pregnancy. Obstet Gynecol Surv 2019; 74:289.

Insulins for Type 2 Diabetes

Original publication date – May 2019

The goal of drug therapy for type 2 diabetes is to achieve and maintain a near-normal glycated hemoglobin (A1C) concentration without inducing hypoglycemia; for most patients, the target A1C is <7%.[1] Metformin is the preferred first-line treatment, but most patients with type 2 diabetes eventually require multidrug therapy and/or insulin to achieve glycemic control.[2]

BASAL INSULIN — When insulin is added to other antihyperglycemic drugs, a basal insulin is usually prescribed first. Available basal insulins include NPH, an intermediate-acting human insulin, and the long-acting insulin analogs (detemir, glargine, and degludec), which are recombinant DNA analogs of human insulin.

NPH insulin *(Humulin N, Novolin N)* has a duration of action of 12 to 24 hours with a peak effect at 4 to 8 hours.

Insulin detemir *(Levemir)* is absorbed slowly from the injection site and is more than 98% reversibly bound to albumin in the blood, further prolonging its duration of action and clearance.[3] The effectiveness of insulin detemir appears to decrease after 12 hours; it may be more effective when used twice daily. In a 26-week trial in 457 patients with type 2 diabetes inadequately controlled on metformin alone, addition of insulin detemir was found to be slightly less effective than addition of insulin glargine in reducing A1C (-0.48% vs -0.74%).[4]

Summary

▸ Basal insulin therapy with a long-acting insulin analog (detemir, glargine, or degludec) is less likely than NPH to cause hypoglycemia.

▸ Mealtime use of regular human insulin or a rapid-acting insulin analog (aspart, glulisine, or lispro) can be added to basal insulin therapy in patients who need further glycemic control.

▸ Rapid-acting insulin analogs are slightly more effective than regular insulin in decreasing A1C, with less hypoglycemia.

▸ Inhaled insulin is rapid-acting but may cause pulmonary problems.

▸ Use of pre-mixed insulin combinations can decrease the number of injections, but dose titration is more difficult and hypoglycemia may occur more often.

▸ The high cost of insulins is a concern. Human insulins are generally available at a lower price than insulin analogs.

Insulin glargine 100 units/mL *(Lantus, Basaglar[5])* forms microprecipitates in subcutaneous tissue, prolonging its duration of action to a mean of 24 hours or longer. It has no pronounced peak effect.

Insulin glargine 300 units/mL *(Toujeo)* has a more gradual and prolonged release of insulin from the subcutaneous depot than *Lantus*, resulting in more even activity throughout the dosing period and a longer duration of action. In clinical trials, insulin glargine 300 units/mL was as effective as insulin glargine 100 units/mL in lowering A1C and in some trials it caused less hypoglycemia.[6] The prolonged time in subcutaneous tissue may, however, reduce its bioavailability. The daily dose of insulin glargine 300 units/mL may need to be 10-15% higher than the dose of insulin glargine 100 units/mL.

Insulin degludec *(Tresiba;* 100 and 200 units/mL) forms multihexamers in subcutaneous tissue, which substantially delays its absorption, and binds to circulating albumin, which delays its elimination, resulting in a duration of action of >42 hours. In clinical trials, insulin degludec 100 units/mL was noninferior to insulin glargine 100 units/mL or insulin detemir in lowering A1C and in some trials caused less hypoglycemia and nocturnal hypoglycemia than insulin glargine.[7,8]

NPH vs Long-Acting Insulin Analogs – Multiple prospective randomized trials have demonstrated similar decreases in A1C with NPH insulin and long-acting insulin analogs and a higher incidence of hypoglycemia, especially nocturnal hypoglycemia, with NPH.[9-12] In recent retrospective observational studies, the rates of serious hypoglycemic events and hypoglycemia-related emergency department visits or hospitalizations were not significantly higher with NPH compared to the long-acting insulin analogs.[13,14] Whether the difference in hypoglycemia rates in prospective trials is clinically significant enough to justify the higher cost of the long-acting insulin analogs is controversial.[15]

Dosage and Administration – In general, when adding a basal insulin (NPH or insulin detemir, glargine, or degludec) to oral or injectable antihyperglycemic drugs, the initial dosage is 10 units per day or 0.1-0.2 units/kg per day, usually injected at bedtime (either the morning or bedtime for glargine or degludec). If fasting hyperglycemia persists, the dose can be increased by 2 units every 3 days to achieve fasting plasma glucose concentrations of 70-130 mg/dL. Twice-daily dosing is usually needed for NPH and insulin detemir, and occasionally for insulin glargine 100 units/mL. NPH can be mixed with rapid-acting insulins (except *Fiasp*); insulins glargine, detemir, and degludec cannot be mixed with other insulins.

PRANDIAL INSULIN — Mealtime use of regular human insulin *(Humulin R, Novolin R)* or a rapid-acting insulin analog can be added to basal insulin therapy in patients who need additional glycemic control. Rapid-acting insulin analogs have a faster onset and shorter duration of action than regular insulin and are generally administered with or just before a meal. Regular insulin is usually injected about 30 minutes before a meal. In general, the rapid-acting insulin analogs **insulin aspart** *(Novolog, Fiasp*[16]*)*, **insulin glulisine** *(Apidra)*, and **insulin lispro** *(Humalog,* and generic, *Admelog*[17]*)* may be slightly more effective than regular insulin in decreasing A1C, with less hypoglycemia.[18-22] There are no significant clinical differences between the three rapid-acting insulin analogs.

Table 1. Some Available Insulins		
Drug	**Concentration**	**Some Formulations**
Intermediate-Acting Insulin		
NPH – *Humulin N*[2] (Lilly)	100 units/mL	3, 10 mL vials
		3 mL *KwikPen*[3]
Novolin N[2] (Novo Nordisk)	100 units/mL	10 mL vials
ReliOn/Novolin N[2]	100 units/mL	10 mL vials
Long-Acting Insulin Analogs		
Insulin detemir – *Levemir* (Novo Nordisk)	100 units/mL	10 mL vials
		3 mL *FlexTouch*[3]
Insulin glargine – *Lantus* (Sanofi)	100 units/mL	10 mL vials
		3 mL *SoloStar*[3]
Basaglar[5] (Lilly)	100 units/mL	3 mL *KwikPen*[3]
Toujeo (Sanofi)	300 units/mL	1.5 mL *SoloStar*[3,7]
		3 mL *Max SoloStar*[3,7]
Insulin degludec – *Tresiba* (Novo Nordisk)	100, 200[9] units/mL	10 mL vials
		3 mL *FlexTouch*[3]
Long-Acting Insulin/GLP-1 Receptor Agonist Combinations		
Insulin glargine/lixisenatide – *Soliqua* (Sanofi)	100 units/33 mcg/mL	3 mL prefilled pens
Insulin degludec/liraglutide – *Xultophy* (Novo Nordisk)	100 units/3.6 mg/mL	3 mL prefilled pens
Rapid-Acting Insulin Analogs		
Insulin aspart – *Novolog* (Novo Nordisk)	100 units/mL	10 mL vials
		3 mL cartridges
		3 mL *FlexPen*[3]
Fiasp[14] (Novo Nordisk)	100 units/mL	10 mL vials
		3 mL *FlexTouch*[3]

1. Approximate WAC for one 10-mL vial or one disposable pen in the lowest available concentration. WAC = wholesaler acquisition cost or manufacturer's published price to wholesalers; WAC represents a published catalogue or list price and may not represent an actual transactional price. Source: Analysource® Monthly. April 5, 2019. Reprinted with permission by First Databank, Inc. All rights reserved. ©2019. www.fdbhealth.com/policies/drug-pricing-policy.
2. Available over the counter.
3. Prefilled, disposable pen. All 100 unit/mL insulin pens are available in boxes containing 5 pens each. *Humalog* 200 units/mL, *Humulin R* 500 units/mL and *Toujeo Max* are available in boxes containing 2 pens each. *Tresiba* 200 units/mL and *Toujeo* are available in boxes containing 3 pens each.
4. Available only at Walmart. Approximate cost for 1 vial.
5. *Basaglar* is a "follow-on" product similar to *Lantus*; it is not interchangeable with *Lantus*.
6. H Linnebjerg et al. Diabetes Obes Metab 2017; 19:33.

Onset	Peak	Duration	Cost[1]
1-2 hrs	4-8 hrs	12-24 hrs	$148.70
			94.30
			137.70
			24.90[4]
1-2 hrs	6-12 hrs	12-24 hrs	308.10
			92.40
1-4 hrs	no peak	~24 hrs	283.60
			85.10
1-4 hrs	no peak	~24 hrs[6]	65.30
1-6 hrs	no peak	24-36 hrs	129.60[8]
1-9 hrs	no peak	>42 hrs	339.00
			101.70[10]
1-4 hrs[11]	no peak	Footnote 12	141.40
1-9 hrs[11]	no peak	Footnote 12	208.00
10-30 mins	1-2 hrs	3-5 hrs	289.40
			107.50[13]
			111.80
~2.5 mins	~63 mins	3-5 hrs	289.40
			111.80

7. The *Toujeo SoloStar* pen contains 450 units of insulin glargine, is adjusted in 1-unit increments, and can deliver up to 80 units per injection. The *Toujeo Max SoloStar* pen contains 900 units of insulin glargine, is adjusted in 2-unit increments, and can deliver up to 160 units per injection.
8. Cost for one *Toujeo SoloStar* 1.5-mL pen.
9. The 100 units/mL strength is available in 10-mL vials and 3-mL pens. The 200 units/mL strength is available in 3-mL pens.
10. Cost for 100 unit/mL pen.
11. Onset of insulin component only.
12. Refer to individual components alone.
13. Cost for one 3-mL cartridge.
14. *Fiasp* is insulin aspart with the addition of two excipients, nicotinamide, which is intended to result in faster initial absorption, and arginine, which increases stability. It is not interchangeable with *Novolog*.

Continued on next page

Table 1. Some Available Insulins (continued)		
Drug	**Concentration**	**Some Formulations**
Rapid-Acting Insulin Analogs (continued)		
Insulin glulisine – *Apidra* (Sanofi)	100 units/mL	10 mL vials 3 mL *SoloStar*[3]
Insulin lispro – generic[15]	100 units/mL	10 mL vials 3 mL *KwikPen*[3]
Humalog (Lilly)	100, 200[16] units/mL	3 mL, 10 mL vials 3 mL cartridges 3 mL *KwikPen*[3]
Admelog[17] (Sanofi)	100 units/mL	3 mL, 10 mL vials 3 mL *SoloStar*[3]
Regular Insulin		
Humulin R (Lilly)	100[2], 500[18] units/mL	3, 10, 20 mL vials[19] 3 mL *KwikPen*[3,19]
Novolin R[2] (Novo Nordisk)	100 units/mL	10 mL vials
ReliOn/Novolin R[2]	100 units/mL	10 mL vials
Insulin inhalation powder – *Afrezza* (Mannkind)	4, 8, 12 units/inh	4, 8, 12 unit cartridges[20]
Pre-Mixed Insulins		
Humalog Mix 75/25[22] (Lilly)	100 units/mL	10 mL vials 3 mL *KwikPen*[3]
Humalog Mix 50/50[23] (Lilly)	100 units/mL	10 mL vials 3 mL *KwikPen*[3]
Novolog Mix 70/30[24] (Novo Nordisk)	100 units/mL	10 mL vials 3 mL *FlexPen*[3]
Humulin 70/30[25] (Lilly)	100 units/mL	10 mL vials 3 mL *KwikPen*[3]
Novolin 70/30[2,25] (Novo Nordisk)	100 units/mL	10 mL vials 3 mL *FlexPen*[3]
ReliOn/Novolin 70/30[2,25] (Novo Nordisk)	100 units/mL	10 mL vials

15. Authorized generic of *Humalog* manufactured by Lilly. Expected to become available in 2019.
16. Only available as a prefilled, disposable pen.
17. *Admelog* is a "follow-on" product similar to *Humalog*; it is not interchangeable with *Humalog*.
18. A dedicated U500 insulin syringe is now available.
19. The 100 units/mL strength is available in 3- and 10-mL vials. The 500 units/mL strength is available in 20-mL vials and 3-mL prefilled pens (*KwikPen*).

Onset	Peak	Duration	Cost[1]
10-30 mins	60 mins	4-5 hrs	$284.00
			109.70
10-30 mins	0.5-2 hrs	3-5 hrs	135.40
			53.00
			274.70
			102.10[13]
			212.20
			233.50
			90.20
30-60 mins	1-5 hrs	4-12 hrs	148.70
			287.10
			137.70
			24.90[4]
12 mins	~35-55 mins	1.5-3 hrs	324.70[21]
5-15 mins	2-4 hrs	14-24 hrs	284.70
			106.10
5-15 mins	2-4 hrs	14-24 hrs	284.70
			106.10
5-15 mins	2-4 hrs	14-24 hrs	300.10
			111.80
30-60 mins	2-12 hrs	12-24 hrs	148.70
			94.30
30-60 mins	2-12 hrs	12-24 hrs	137.70
			52.10
			24.90[4]

20. Administered via breath-powered inhaler.
21. Cost for one package containing 90 4-unit cartridges of *Afrezza* and 2 inhalers.
22. 75% insulin lispro protamine suspension and 25% insulin lispro injection.
23. 50% insulin lispro protamine suspension and 50% insulin lispro injection.
24. 70% insulin aspart protamine suspension and 30% insulin aspart injection.
25. 70% NPH, human insulin isophane suspension and 30% regular human insulin injection.

An inhaled, rapid-acting, dry-powder formulation of recombinant regular human insulin *(Afrezza)* reaches peak concentrations more rapidly than insulin lispro.[23] It should not be used in patients who smoke or in patients with lung cancer and is contraindicated for use in patients with chronic lung disease such as asthma or COPD; pulmonary function testing should be performed before starting *Afrezza*. The dose of *Afrezza* can only be adjusted in 4-unit increments.

Dosage and Administration – Patients who are unable to achieve glycemic goals on basal insulin can start a prandial insulin with a dose of 2-4 units per day or 10% of the basal dose given with the largest meal or the meal with the largest postprandial glucose excursion. A reduction in the basal insulin dose may be needed in some patients.

Regular insulin is most effective when taken about 30 minutes before a meal. The rapid-acting analogs are generally effective when taken within 15 minutes of a meal. Inhaled insulin is administered at the beginning of a meal.

PRE-MIXED COMBINATIONS — Use of pre-mixed insulin combinations simplifies administration, but dose titration is more difficult and hypoglycemia may be more frequent than with individual insulins. They are not recommended for insulin-naive patients.

LONG-ACTING INSULIN/GLP-1 RECEPTOR AGONIST COMBINATIONS — *Soliqua*, a fixed-ratio combination of insulin glargine and the GLP-1 receptor agonist lixisenatide, and *Xultophy*, a fixed-ratio combination of insulin degludec and the GLP-1 receptor agonist liraglutide, are FDA-approved for treatment of type 2 diabetes.[24,25] They reduce A1C more than their individual components alone and may improve adherence.

ADVERSE EFFECTS — All insulins, including long-acting formulations, can cause hypoglycemia and weight gain. Other adverse effects include allergic reactions, injection-site reactions, lipodystrophy, pruritus, rash, and edema.

Transient cough and throat pain are common with use of **inhaled insulin**. An average decrease in FEV_1 of 40 mL has been reported in clinical trials lasting up to 2 years; patients with chronic lung disease were excluded from these trials. Acute bronchospasm has occurred in patients with asthma or COPD.

PREGNANCY AND LACTATION — Insulin is the drug of choice for treatment of pregnant women with type 2 diabetes that is not adequately controlled with diet and exercise.[1] Insulin is a normal component of human breast milk and adequate glycemic control is needed for milk production. Women taking exogenous insulin, which passes into breast milk, can breastfeed.

COST — The high cost of insulins has become a significant issue.[15] Most costs listed in Table 1 represent the wholesaler acquisition cost (WAC) or the manufacturer's published price to wholesalers for a single vial or prefilled pen, which is not enough to last one month for most patients. Patients with no insurance or those who are underinsured may pay the WAC price or more. Regular human insulin, NPH insulin, and a pre-mixed combination are available in 10-mL vials at Walmart for $24.90 per vial.

1. American Diabetes Association. Standards of medical care in diabetes – 2019. Diabetes Care 2019; 42 (Suppl):S1.
2. Drugs for type 2 diabetes. Med Lett Drugs Ther 2017; 59:9.
3. Insulin detemir (Levemir), a new long-acting insulin. Med Lett Drugs Ther 2006; 48:54.
4. L Meneghini et al. Once-daily initiation of basal insulin as add-on to metformin: a 26-week, randomized, treat-to-target trial comparing insulin detemir with insulin glargine in patients with type 2 diabetes. Diabetes Obes Metab 2013; 15:729.
5. Another insulin glargine (Basaglar) for diabetes. Med Lett Drugs Ther 2017; 59:3.
6. Concentrated insulin glargine (Toujeo) for diabetes. Med Lett Drugs Ther 2015; 57:69.
7. Insulin degludec (Tresiba) – a new long-acting insulin for diabetes. Med Lett Drugs Ther 2015; 57:163.

8. C Wysham et al. Effect of insulin degludec vs insulin glargine U100 on hypoglycemia in patients with type 2 diabetes: the SWITCH 2 randomized clinical trial. JAMA 2017: 318:45.

9. MC Riddle et al. The treat-to-target trial: randomized addition of glargine or human NPH insulin to oral therapy of type 2 diabetic patients. Diabetes Care 2003; 26:3080.

10. J Rosenstock et al. Similar progression of diabetic retinopathy with insulin glargine and neutral protamine Hagedorn (NPH) insulin in patients with type 2 diabetes: a long-term, randomised, open-label study. Diabetologia 2009; 52:1778.

11. K Horvath et al. Long-acting insulin analogues versus NPH insulin (human isophane insulin) for type 2 diabetes mellitus (review). Cochrane Database Syst Rev 2007; 2:CD005613.

12. K Hermansen et al. A 26-week, randomized, parallel, treat-to-target trial comparing insulin detemir with NPH insulin as add-on therapy to oral glucose-lowering drugs in insulin-naive people with type 2 diabetes. Diabetes Care 2006; 29:1269.

13. KJ Lipska et al. Association of initiation of basal insulin analogs vs neutral protamine Hagedorn (NPH) insulin with hypoglycemia-related emergency department visits or hospital admissions and with glycemic control in patients with type 2 diabetes. JAMA 2018; 320:53.

14. J Luo et al. Implementation of a health plan program for switching from analogue to human insulin and glycemic control among Medicare beneficiaries with type 2 diabetes. JAMA 2019; 321:374.

15. KJ Lipska et al. Insulin analogues for type 2 diabetes. JAMA 2019; 321:350.

16. Fiasp - another insulin aspart formulation for diabetes. Med Lett Drugs Ther 2018; 60:6.

17. In brief: another insulin lispro (Admelog) for diabetes. Med Lett Drugs Ther 2018; 60:e109.

18. SR Singh et al. Efficacy and safety of insulin analogues for the management of diabetes mellitus: a meta-analysis. CMAJ 2009; 180:385.

19. Rapid-acting insulin analogs. Med Lett Drugs Ther 2009; 51:98.

20. Insulin glulisine (Apidra): a new rapid-acting insulin. Med Lett Drugs Ther 2006; 48:33.

21. E Mannucci et al. Short-acting insulin analogues vs. regular human insulin in type 2 diabetes: a meta-analysis. Diabetes Obes Metab 2009; 11:53.

22. S Heller et al. Meta-analysis of insulin aspart versus regular human insulin used in a basal-bolus regimen for the treatment of diabetes mellitus. J Diabetes 2013; 5:482.

23. An inhaled insulin (Afrezza). Med Lett Drugs Ther 2015; 57:34.

24. Insulin degludec/liraglutide (Xultophy 100/3.6) for type 2 diabetes. Med Lett Drugs Ther 2017; 59:147.

25. Lixisenatide for type 2 diabetes. Med Lett Drugs Ther 2017; 59:19.

DRUGS FOR
Common Eye Disorders

Original publication date – December 2019

This issue includes reviews of drugs for glaucoma, age-related macular degeneration (AMD), bacterial conjunctivitis, and dry eye disease. Allergic conjunctivitis is reviewed in a separate issue.[1]

In general, all eye drops should be given in doses of one drop. The average volume of a single drop is larger than the eyelid's capacity to hold fluid; a second drop only washes out the first, may increase systemic absorption, and doubles the cost of treatment. The interval between instillation of 2 different drops should be at least 5 minutes. Patients who experience stinging or burning following application of a topical ophthalmic product should try refrigerating the product before use.

GLAUCOMA

Glaucoma is a progressive optic neuropathy often associated with increased intraocular pressure (IOP; normal range 8-22 mm Hg), which is the only disease-related effect that can be modified. Treatment of open-angle glaucoma in adults is reviewed here. Topical drugs are listed in Table 1; laser trabeculoplasty and surgery are alternatives to medication.

PROSTAGLANDIN ANALOGS — Topical prostaglandin analogs (PGAs) are the drugs of choice for initial treatment of open-angle glaucoma. PGAs increase uveoscleral outflow; they have a lesser effect on

Summary

Glaucoma

▶ Topical drugs that lower intraocular pressure (IOP) are the mainstay of treatment for open-angle glaucoma; laser trabeculoplasty and surgery are alternatives.
▶ Topical prostaglandin analog (PGA) monotherapy is preferred for initial treatment.
▶ A topical beta blocker, carbonic anhydrase inhibitor, selective alpha$_2$-agonist, or netarsudil could be added or substituted if IOP fails to reach the target range (8-22 mm Hg).

Age-Related Macular Degeneration (AMD)

▶ A formulation of antioxidant vitamins and zinc is often recommended to prevent progression from dry to wet AMD; its efficacy is unclear.
▶ Treatment of wet AMD with VEGF inhibitors has reduced vision loss in many patients and has recovered lost vision in patients whose treatment began soon after the onset of leakage.

Bacterial Conjunctivitis

▶ Erythromycin ophthalmic ointment or trimethoprim/polymyxin B ophthalmic solution would be a reasonable choice for first-line treatment of bacterial conjunctivitis.
▶ Alternatives include bacitracin or bacitracin/polymyxin B, azithromycin, and a topical fluoroquinolone.
▶ In contact lens wearers, who have a higher incidence of pseudomonal infection, a topical fluoroquinolone is preferred.

Dry Eye Disease

▶ Artificial tear solutions or ointments are the most cost-effective options for initial treatment of dry eye disease.
▶ The daily ocular insert *Lacrisert* is indicated for treatment of moderate to severe dry eye syndromes.
▶ Topical cyclosporine formulations (*Restasis, Cequa*) appear to be safe and effective, but may take 4-6 weeks to achieve results.
▶ Lifitegrast (*Xiidra*) appears to be safe and modestly effective, but how it compares to other products remains to be determined.

outflow through the trabecular network. Dosed once daily, usually at night, they typically lower IOP by 25-30%.

Adverse Effects – PGAs are generally well tolerated and have few, if any, systemic adverse effects. They can cause conjunctival hyperemia and, with long-term use, irreversible darkening of the iris in people with multicolor irides (green-brown, yellow-brown, or blue/gray-brown), increases in the length, thickness, and darkness of eyelashes, and an increase in periorbital skin pigmentation. PGAs may also cause local irritation, itching, dryness, blurred vision, and periorbital fat atrophy, which leads to deepening of the eyelid sulcus. They rarely cause uveitis or cystoid macular edema.

BETA BLOCKERS — Topical beta blockers decrease aqueous humor production. They lower IOP by 20-25% with once- or twice-daily dosing. The selective beta$_1$-blocker betaxolol (*Betoptic S*, and generics) may cause fewer systemic adverse effects than nonselective beta blockers, but it is less effective at lowering IOP.

Adverse Effects – Topical beta blockers are generally well tolerated; they may rarely cause stinging, itching, redness, and blurred vision. Systemic adverse effects include fatigue, dizziness, bradycardia, respiratory depression, and masking of hypoglycemia. These drugs can block the effects of inhaled beta$_2$-agonists used to treat asthma. Topical beta blockers should be used with caution in patients with bradycardia, asthma, or chronic obstructive pulmonary disease.

CARBONIC ANHYDRASE INHIBITORS — Carbonic anhydrase inhibitors (CAIs), like beta blockers, lower IOP by decreasing production of aqueous humor. Oral CAIs such as acetazolamide or methazolamide can decrease IOP by 30-50%, but have many systemic adverse effects. The topical CAIs dorzolamide (*Trusopt*, and generics) and brinzolamide *(Azopt)* typically lower IOP by 15-20%. Topical CAIs are FDA-approved for use three times daily, but twice-daily use is often effective.

Adverse Effects – Topical CAIs can cause stinging, redness, burning, conjunctivitis, dry eyes, and blurred vision. Generally their only systemic adverse effect has been bitter taste. Although CAIs are sulfonamide derivatives, topical formulations have been well tolerated in most patients with sulfonamide allergies.

Table 1. Some Topical Drugs for Glaucoma

Drug	Some Formulations
Prostaglandin Analogs (PGAs)	
Bimatoprost – *Lumigan* (Allergan)	0.01% soln*
Latanoprost – *Xalatan* (Pfizer) generic	0.005% soln*
Xelpros (Sun)	0.005% emulsion
Latanoprostene bunod – *Vyzulta* (Bausch + Lomb)	0.024% soln*
Tafluprost – *Zioptan* (Merck)	0.0015% soln
Travoprost – *Travatan Z* (Alcon)	0.004% soln*
Beta Blockers	
Betaxolol[3] – generic	0.5% soln*
Betoptic S (Alcon)	0.25% susp*
Carteolol – generic	1% soln*
Levobunolol – generic	0.5% soln*
Metipranolol – generic	0.3% soln*
Timolol – *Timoptic* (Bausch + Lomb) generic	0.25%, 0.5% soln*
Timoptic Ocudose	0.25%, 0.5% soln
Timoptic-XE generic	0.25%, 0.5% soln, gel forming
Istalol (Bausch + Lomb)	0.5% soln*
Betimol (Vistakon)	0.25%, 0.5% soln*
Carbonic Anhydrase Inhibitors (CAIs)	
Brinzolamide – *Azopt* (Alcon)	1% susp*
Dorzolamide – *Trusopt* (Merck) generic	2% soln*
Alpha$_2$-Agonists	
Apraclonidine – generic	0.5% soln*
Iopidine (Alcon)	1% soln*

*Contains the preservative benzalkonium chloride, which may cause irritation.
1. Approximate WAC for the smallest size bottle of the lowest available strength. WAC = wholesaler acquisition cost or manufacturer's published price to wholesalers; WAC represents a published catalogue or list price and may not represent an actual transactional price. Source: AnalySource® Monthly. November 5, 2019. Reprinted with permission by First Databank, Inc. All rights reserved. ©2019. www.fdbhealth.com/policies/drug-pricing-policy.

Some Available Sizes	Usual Daily Dosage	Cost[1]
2.5, 5, 7.5 mL	1 drop qPM	$197.00
2.5 mL	1 drop qPM	203.80
		12.30
		55.00
2.5, 5 mL	1 drop qPM	190.80
0.3 mL individual units	1 drop qPM	213.00[2]
2.5, 5 mL	1 drop qPM	183.90
5, 10, 15 mL	1 drop qAM or bid	50.90
10, 15 mL		310.50
5, 10, 15 mL	1 drop qAM or bid	13.00
5, 10, 15 mL	1 drop qAM or bid	11.30
5 mL	1 drop qAM or bid	20.80
5, 10 mL	1 drop bid	174.00
5, 10, 15 mL		4.40
0.2 mL individual units		418.30[4]
5 mL	1 drop once/day	203.60
		165.20
2.5, 5 mL	1 drop qAM	172.40
5, 10, 15 mL[5]	1 drop bid	127.80
10, 15 mL	1 drop bid or tid	308.40
10 mL	1 drop bid or tid	75.80
		34.30
5, 10 mL	1 drop bid or tid	67.50
0.1 mL individual units		665.50[6]

2. Cost of 30 single-use containers.
3. Betaxolol is beta-1 selective.
4. Cost of 60 single-use containers.
5. The 0.25% solution is only available in a 5-mL size.
6. Cost of 24 single-use containers.

Continued on next page

Table 1. Some Topical Drugs for Glaucoma (continued)	
Drug	**Some Formulations**
Alpha₂-Agonists (continued)	
Brimonidine – generic	0.2% soln*
Alphagan P (Allergan)	0.1%, 0.15% soln
generic	0.15% soln
Rho Kinase Inhibitor	
Netarsudil – *Rhopressa* (Aerie)	0.02% soln*
Combinations	
Brinzolamide/brimonidine – *Simbrinza* (Alcon)	1%/0.2% soln*
Brimonidine/timolol – *Combigan* (Allergan)	0.2%/0.5% soln*
Netarsudil/latanoprost – *Rocklatan* (Aerie)	0.2%/0.005% soln*
Timolol/dorzolamide – *Cosopt* (Merck)	0.5%/2% soln*
generic	
Cosopt PF	0.5%/2% soln
generic	
*Contains the preservative benzalkonium chloride, which may cause irritation.	

ALPHA AGONISTS — Like beta blockers and CAIs, alpha agonists lower IOP by decreasing aqueous humor production, but they also increase uveoscleral outflow. The selective alpha₂-agonist brimonidine (*Alphagan P*, and generics) typically lowers IOP by 15-20%.[2] Apraclonidine (*Iopidine,* and generics), a derivative of clonidine, is sometimes used to prevent acute increases in IOP after laser procedures; tachyphylaxis and local allergic reactions have limited its use for long-term IOP control.[3]

Adverse Effects – Local adverse effects of alpha agonists include stinging, conjunctival hyperemia, foreign-body sensation, and dry eyes. The tolerability of brimonidine may be improved by use of a formulation that does not contain the preservative benzalkonium chloride and use of the lower concentration (0.1% vs 0.15%). Fatigue, somnolence, and local allergic reactions occur frequently with use of topical alpha agonists. Brimonidine can cross the blood-brain barrier and cause

Some Available Sizes	Usual Daily Dosage	Cost[1]
5, 10, 15 mL	1 drop bid or tid	$14.80
		160.00
		140.20
2.5 mL	1 drop qPM	272.10
8 mL	1 drop tid	162.70
5, 10, 15 mL	1 drop bid	176.30
2.5 mL	1 drop qPM	285.20
10 mL	1 drop bid	209.60
		50.00
0.2 mL individual units		165.60[4]
		135.60[4]

systemic hypotension in infants and children; it has caused respiratory depression in children <2 years old and should not be used in children <6 years old. Alpha agonists are contraindicated for use in patients taking a monoamine oxidase (MAO) inhibitor.

RHO KINASE INHIBITOR — Netarsudil *(Rhopressa)*, the only Rho kinase inhibitor approved in the US, decreases resistance in the trabecular network outflow pathway. In clinical trials, it was as effective as timolol in patients with a baseline IOP of <25 mm Hg, but did not meet the criteria for noninferiority compared to latanoprost.[4]

Adverse Effects – In clinical trials of netarsudil, about 50% of patients developed conjunctival hyperemia and about 20% developed corneal verticillata (corneal deposits forming a golden brown or gray whorl pattern in the inferior cornea; most resolved when treatment was discontinued). Instillation-site pain, erythema, conjunctival hemorrhage, corneal staining, blurred vision, increased lacrimation, eyelid erythema, and reduced visual acuity were also reported.[4]

CHOLINERGIC AGONISTS — Stimulation of muscarinic receptors by cholinergic agonists causes contraction of the ciliary muscle, leading to an increase in outflow of aqueous humor and a decrease in IOP. Pilocarpine mimics the effect of acetylcholine.

Adverse Effects – Topical application of cholinergic agonists can cause local and systemic adverse effects that limit their use. Contraction of the ciliary muscle leads to ciliary spasm and resulting brow ache. Corneal toxicity, conjunctival inflammation, transient myopia, and blurred vision can occur. Retinal detachment can also occur, especially in highly myopic patients. Systemic adverse effects are rare at recommended doses, but can include sweating, nausea, salivation, and changes in blood pressure. In cases of systemic toxicity, atropine can be used to reverse the symptoms.

COMBINATIONS — Combination products can produce a greater reduction in IOP than monotherapy, but their adverse effects are additive as well. They may be helpful in promoting adherence in patients who require treatment with two drug classes.

MARIJUANA — Use of marijuana can lower IOP by about 25% in patients with or without glaucoma. The mechanism of action is not clear, but may be related to a marijuana-induced decrease in blood pressure. Cannabidiol does not have an IOP-lowering effect.[5,6] Marijuana has a short duration of action (3-4 hours); the adverse cognitive effects of the 6-8 daily doses that would be required to achieve a sustained decrease in IOP should limit its use.[7]

CHOICE OF DRUGS — Topical drugs that lower IOP are the mainstay of treatment for open-angle glaucoma. For initial treatment, PGA monotherapy is preferred; if the PGA lowers IOP into the target range, no additional treatment is necessary. If it substantially decreases IOP, but falls short of achieving the target range, another agent such as a topical beta blocker, a topical CAI, a selective alpha$_2$-agonist, or netarsudil could be added. If the PGA fails to lower IOP substantially, it should be stopped and another drug substituted. Some patients who do not respond to one PGA may respond to another.

LASER TRABECULOPLASTY — Laser trabeculoplasty, a painless outpatient procedure, increases aqueous outflow through the trabecular membrane. Selective laser trabeculoplasty (SLT) has been as effective as argon laser trabeculoplasty in lowering IOP and is better tolerated; transient inflammation of the anterior chamber and spikes in IOP can occur. SLT causes less damage to the trabecular membrane than the argon laser and can be repeated, which may be necessary because its IOP-lowering effect decreases over time. SLT may be less effective when used after topical therapy.[8] In a large randomized controlled trial in previously untreated patients with glaucoma, SLT was as effective as eye drops, less expensive, and better tolerated (one spike in IOP that required treatment out of 776 procedures).[9]

SURGERY — Many different surgical procedures have been used to lower IOP. Risks of surgery include scarring of the eye, cataract formation, and permanent vision loss. Newer, minimally invasive surgical techniques may reduce these risks.[10]

AGE-RELATED MACULAR DEGENERATION

Age-related macular degeneration (AMD) has two major forms. The dry or non-neovascular form is characterized by abnormalities of the retinal pigment epithelium with focal accumulation of metabolic byproducts known as drusen. About 90% of patients with AMD have the dry form; they may experience a slow reduction in central vision. There is no established treatment for dry AMD. The wet or neovascular form, characterized by an often rapid decrease in central visual acuity due to newly developed leaky vessels growing from the choroid into the subretinal

Table 2. VEGF Inhibitors for Neovascular AMD			
Drug	Formulations	Intravitreal Dosage	Cost[1]
Aflibercept – Eylea (Regeneron)	2 mg/0.05 mL single-use vials	2 mg q4 wks x 3 doses, then q8 wks	$1850.00
Bevacizumab[2] – Avastin (Genentech) MVASI (Amgen)	25 mg/mL; 4, 16 mL vials	1.25 mg q4 wks	50.00[3]
Brolucizumab – Beovu (Novartis)	6 mg/0.05 mL single-use vials	6 mg q4 wks x 3 doses, then q8-12 wks	1850.00
Pegaptanib sodium – Macugen (Bausch + Lomb)	0.3 mg/0.09 mL single-use syringes	0.3 mg q6 wks	741.00
Ranibizumab – Lucentis (Genentech)	0.3 mg/0.05 mL, 0.5 mg/0.05 mL single-use vials	0.5 mg q4 wks	1170.00

1. Approximate WAC for one intravitreal injection (administration cost not included). WAC = wholesaler acquisition cost or manufacturer's published price to wholesalers; WAC represents a published catalogue or list price and may not represent an actual transactional price. Source: AnalySource® Monthly. November 5, 2019. Reprinted with permission by First Databank, Inc. All rights reserved. ©2019. www.fdbhealth.com/policies/drug-pricing-policy.
2. Not FDA-approved for treatment of AMD.
3. Cost of a 4-mL single-use vial of Avastin is $796.94 and of MVASI is $677.40. A compounding pharmacy can divide the vial into small aliquots. Actual retail prices may vary.

space, occurs in about 10% of patients. More than 90% of AMD-related vision loss in the US is caused by wet AMD.

ANTIOXIDANTS AND ZINC — Various oral vitamin supplements are promoted for ocular health and specifically for AMD. Antioxidants have been theorized to decrease inflammation and perhaps reduce oxidative stress caused by metabolic byproducts in and around the retina.

AREDS — In the Age-Related Eye Disease Study (AREDS), a double-masked prospective study sponsored by the National Eye Institute and Bausch + Lomb, 3640 patients 55-80 years old with various stages of AMD were randomized to receive one of four treatments: antioxidants at doses 5-15 times higher than the recommended dietary allowance (vitamin C 500 mg, vitamin E 400 IU, and beta carotene 15 mg), zinc (80 mg of zinc as zinc oxide and 2 mg of copper as cupric oxide), antioxidants plus zinc, or placebo. The primary endpoints were progression to advanced AMD (choroidal neovascularization or geographic atrophy including the center of the macula) and moderate loss of visual acuity (3 or more lines of vision).

After 5 years of treatment, no benefit was seen in 1063 patients who joined the study with only multiple small or a few medium drusen and good vision in the eye with more advanced disease. When these patients were excluded from the analysis (a post-hoc analysis), the estimated probability of progression to advanced AMD among the remaining patients was 28% with placebo, 23% with antioxidants alone, 22% with zinc alone, and 20% with antioxidants plus zinc. Only the combination of antioxidants and zinc had a statistically significant effect compared to placebo.[11]

A Second Study – AREDS2 was limited to patients with bilateral intermediate AMD or intermediate AMD in one eye and advanced AMD in the other eye. The design was complex: patients were randomized to receive lutein plus zeaxanthin, docosahexaenoic acid (DHA) plus eicosapentaenoic acid (EPA), both, or placebo, all in addition to the original AREDS formulation. Participants were also offered a secondary randomization to one of four variations of the original AREDS formula that included lower doses of zinc, omission of beta carotene, or both. There was no true placebo group; all participants received the original AREDS formulation or some variation of it.

The 5-year probability of progression to advanced AMD was found to be nearly identical (29%-31%) in all groups. The only significant finding was that lung cancers occurred more frequently in patients who received beta carotene than in those who did not (2% vs 0.9%).[12]

Adverse Effects – In 2 prospective double-blind trials, long-term use (4-8 years) of a high dose (20 mg) of beta carotene in male smokers resulted in an increased incidence of lung cancer and death beginning 18 months after starting treatment.[13,14] Some studies have suggested that vitamin E, particularly in doses >400 mg/day, may increase all-cause mortality.[15,16]

VEGF INHIBITORS — The principal mediator of neovascularization in wet AMD is thought to be vascular endothelial growth factor (VEGF), which induces angiogenesis and increases vascular permeability. Treatment of wet AMD with VEGF inhibitors has reduced vision loss in many patients and has recovered lost vision in patients whose treatment began soon after the onset of leakage. These drugs are given as periodic intravitreal injections with topical anesthesia. They can cause ocular inflammation, increased IOP and, rarely, serious complications such as retinal detachment and endophthalmitis, leading to loss of vision.[17]

Ranibizumab *(Lucentis)* – FDA-approved for wet AMD,[18] ranibizumab is also approved for treatment of diabetic macular edema (DME), retinal vein occlusion, and diabetic retinopathy. Ranibizumab is a recombinant, humanized monoclonal antibody fragment (Fab) derived from the same antibody as bevacizumab that causes regression of the abnormal vessels and reduction of leakage from these vessels in wet AMD, improves visual acuity, and decreases swelling of the retina.

In one controlled trial (MARINA) in AMD patients, 95% of patients who received monthly injections of ranibizumab 0.3 or 0.5 mg for one year lost fewer than 15 letters of visual acuity, compared to 62% of those who received sham injections. Visual acuity improved by 15 or more letters in 25% and 34% of patients injected with ranibizumab 0.3 mg and 0.5 mg, respectively, compared to 5% of those who received sham injections. At 1 year, the average gain from baseline was 6.5 letters with ranibizumab 0.3 mg and 7.2 letters with ranibizumab 0.5 mg, compared to a loss of 10.4 letters with sham injections. The average gain in visual acuity was maintained at 2 years with continued treatment: 6.6 letters gained (with 0.5 mg) vs 14.9 letters lost (with sham injections).[19]

Bevacizumab *(Avastin, MVASI)* – FDA-approved for treatment of metastatic colorectal cancer and other advanced cancers, bevacizumab has been used off-label for treatment of wet AMD. Divided into aliquots, it costs much less than pegaptanib or ranibizumab, but repackaging of the drug without proper aseptic technique has led to endophthalmitis in a small number of patients.[20] An NIH-sponsored trial (CATT) and a parallel UK trial (IVAN) comparing monthly or as-needed injections of bevacizumab with ranibizumab found equivalent effects on visual acuity after 1 and 2 years (8 and 18.4 letters gained with bevacizumab vs 8.5 and 17.0 letters gained with ranibizumab).[21,22] Patients who were randomized from monthly to as-needed treatment with either drug after 1 year had a mean decrease in vision during the second year.[23]

Aflibercept *(Eylea)* – A fusion protein FDA-approved for treatment of wet AMD, aflibercept acts as a decoy VEGF receptor, competing for binding of VEGF. Aflibercept is also approved for treatment of diabetic macular edema, macular edema following retinal vein occlusion, and diabetic retinopathy. In 2 controlled trials, it appeared to be similar to ranibizumab in effectiveness.[24] Aflibercept has not been compared directly to bevacizumab.

Brolucizumab *(Beovu)* – Recently approved by the FDA for treatment of wet AMD, brolucizumab is dosed every 8-12 weeks (after a 3-month loading phase). In 2 randomized, double-blind trials, it was noninferior to aflibercept in visual function at week 48, and similar in safety.[25] It has not been compared to ranibizumab or bevacizumab.

Pegaptanib sodium *(Macugen)* – Pegaptanib was the first VEGF inhibitor approved by the FDA for treatment of wet AMD.[26] It appears to be less effective than ranibizumab or bevacizumab and has not been shown to improve vision.[27]

Adverse Effects – The adverse effects of VEGF inhibitors have been largely related to the procedure rather than the drug itself; they include conjunctival hemorrhage, acute IOP rise after injection, traumatic cataract, uveitis, and retinal detachment, all occurring in less than 2% of patients. Intravitreal injection of VEGF inhibitors carries a risk of intraocular infection and endophthalmitis. In one study, endophthalmitis developed after 2 of 5449 ranibizumab injections (0.04%) and after 4 of 5508 bevacizumab injections (0.07%).[21]

PHOTODYNAMIC THERAPY — Verteporfin *(Visudyne)* is a benzo-porphyrin derivative that is infused intravenously. Activated in the eye by low-intensity infrared light 15 minutes following infusion, it occludes abnormal blood vessels while (relatively) sparing normal vessels and tissue. However, the visual outcome in eyes treated with photodynamic therapy is generally not as good as in eyes treated with VEGF inhibitors.[28]

A meta-analysis comparing anti-VEGF monotherapy with combined anti-VEGF therapy and verteporfin photodynamic therapy found no difference in best corrected visual acuity (BCVA), central retinal thick-ness, or the proportion of patients who gained >15 BCVA letters. Patients treated with the combination required fewer anti-VEGF injections than those who received monotherapy.[29]

Adverse Effects – A sudden severe decrease in visual acuity, usually transient and probably caused by post-treatment swelling, has been reported in <5% of patients who received photodynamic therapy. Tran-sient back pain occurs in about 2% of patients during the infusion. The skin and eyes of patients who receive verteporfin may be sensitive to sunlight and high-intensity halogen lights for up to 5 days after the infu-sion. Patients with porphyria should not receive photodynamic therapy.

CHOICE OF DRUGS — Whether any drug can slow the progression of dry AMD is unclear. For treatment of wet AMD, ranibizumab, beva-cizumab, aflibercept, and brolucizumab can reduce vision loss in many patients and can recover lost vision in patients whose treatment began soon after the onset of leakage. Bevacizumab used off-label costs much less than VEGF inhibitors that are FDA-approved for treatment of wet AMD, and it appears to be as effective as ranibizumab. Aflibercept also appears to be as effective as ranibizumab; it has not been compared directly with bevacizumab. Brolucizumab is dosed less frequently than other anti-VEGF drugs and has been shown to be noninferior to aflibercept, but how it compares to ranibizumab or bevacizumab remains to be determined.

BACTERIAL CONJUNCTIVITIS

In the US, the most common bacterial pathogen associated with acute conjunctivitis in adults is *Staphylococcus aureus. Streptococcus pneumoniae, Haemophilus influenzae, and Moraxella catarrhalis* are common pathogens in children.[30] Ophthalmic administration of antibacterials is much less likely to cause adverse effects than systemic administration.

OPHTHALMIC ANTIBACTERIALS — Ophthalmic formulations of antibacterial drugs achieve high concentrations on the surface of the eye and can be effective in treating surface ocular infections, even when the organisms are reported to be resistant *in vitro*. **Sulfacetamide** is not highly effective, can be sensitizing, and rarely has caused Stevens-Johnson syndrome. **Neomycin** causes sensitization and other local adverse reactions in about 5-10% of patients. **Bacitracin** and **erythromycin** are not active against the gram-negative organisms that cause a small percentage of acute conjunctival infections in adults. **Polymyxin B** is only active against gram-negative organisms. **Trimethoprim** has a broad spectrum of activity, often including methicillin-resistant staphylococci. Ophthalmic **azithromycin**[31] has activity primarily against gram-positive microbes, but also against *H. influenzae*. A single oral dose of azithromycin is effective for treatment of *Chlamydia trachomatis* and gonococcal conjunctivitis. All **fluoroquinolones** are active against most bacteria associated with conjunctivitis. *S. aureus* and some anaerobes that are resistant *in vitro* to older fluoroquinolones such as ciprofloxacin and ofloxacin may be susceptible to moxifloxacin, gatifloxacin, and besifloxacin.[32]

CHOICE OF OPHTHALMIC DRUGS — Erythromycin ophthalmic ointment or trimethoprim/polymyxin B ophthalmic solution would be a reasonable choice for first-line treatment of acute bacterial conjunctivitis; alternatives include bacitracin or bacitracin/polymyxin B ointment, azithromycin, or a topical fluoroquinolone (see Table 3). In contact lens

Table 3. Some Ophthalmic Antimicrobials for Bacterial Conjunctivitis

Drug	Formulations
Fluoroquinolones	
Besifloxacin – *Besivance* (Bausch + Lomb)	0.6% susp
Ciprofloxacin – generic	0.3% soln
Ciloxan (Alcon)	0.3% soln
	0.3% oint
Gatifloxacin – generic	0.5% soln
Zymaxid (Allergan)	0.5% soln
Levofloxacin – generic	0.5% soln
Moxifloxacin – generic	0.5% soln
Vigamox (Alcon)	0.5% soln
Moxeza (Alcon)[4]	0.5% soln
Ofloxacin – generic	0.3% soln
Ocuflox (Allergan)	0.3% soln
Other Single Agents	
Azithromycin – *Azasite* (Inspire)	1% soln
Erythromycin – generic	0.5% oint
Gentamicin – generic	0.3% soln
Gentak (Akorn)	0.3% oint
Sulfacetamide sodium – generic	10% oint
	10% soln
Bleph-10 (Allergan)	10% soln
Tobramycin – generic	0.3% soln
Tobrex (Alcon)	0.3% soln
	0.3% oint

susp = suspension; soln = solution; oint = ointment
1. Wholesale acquisition cost (WAC) for the smallest size tube or bottle available. WAC = wholesaler acquisition cost or manufacturer's published price to wholesalers; WAC represents a published catalogue or list price and may not represent an actual transactional price. Source: AnalySource® Monthly. November 5, 2019. Reprinted with permission by First Databank, Inc. All rights reserved. ©2019. www.fdbhealth.com/policies/drug-pricing-policy.

Some Available Sizes	Usual Dosage	Cost[1]
5 mL	1 drop q8h x 7 days[2,3]	$169.40
2.5, 5, 10 mL	1-2 drops q2h x 2 days, then 1-2 drops q4h x	9.80
5 mL	5 days[3]	120.90
3.5 g	0.5 inch q8h x 3 days, then 0.5 inch q12h x	214.40
	5 days[3]	
2.5 mL	1 drop q2h (max 8 doses) x 1 day, then 1 drop	94.50
2.5 mL	q6-12h x 6 days[3]	175.00
5 mL	1-2 drops q2h (max 8 doses) x 2 days, then 1-2	79.50
	drops q4h (max 4 doses) x 5 days[3]	
3 mL	1 drop q8h x 7 days	82.50
3 mL		174.10
3 mL	1 drop q12h x 7 days	169.70
5, 10 mL	1-2 drops q2-4h x 2 days, then 1-2 drops q6h	53.00
5 mL	x 5 days	118.20
2.5 mL	1 drop q12h x 2 days, then 1 drop once/day x	206.20
	5 days	
1, 3.5 g	0.5 inch q6h x 5-7 days	8.40
5 mL	1-2 drops q4h x 7 days	17.70
3.5 g	0.5 inch q8-12h x 7 days	28.40
3.5 g	0.5 inch q3-4h x 7-10 days[5]	54.90
5, 15 mL	1-2 drops q2-3h x 7-10 days[5]	31.30
5 mL		133.00
5 mL	1-2 drops q4h x 7 days[6]	13.20
5 mL		102.10
3.5 g	0.5 inch q8-12h x 7 days[6]	214.40

2. Doses should be 4-12 hours apart.
3. While awake.
4. Contains the same active agent as *Vigamox*, but has a different vehicle (xanthum gum).
5. Dosage may be tapered by increasing time interval between doses as the condition responds.
6. For mild to moderate infections. For severe infections, dosage is 2 drops/h or 0.5 inch q3-4h until improvement; dosage should be reduced prior to discontinuation.

Continued on next page

Table 3. Some Ophthalmic Antimicrobials for Bacterial Conjunctivitis (continued)	
Drug	**Formulations**
Combinations	
Polymyxin B/bacitracin − generic	oint
Polymyxin B/neomycin/bacitracin − generic	oint
Polymyxin B/neomycin/gramicidin − generic	soln
Polymyxin B/trimethoprim − generic	soln
Polytrim (Allergan)	soln
soln = solution; oint = ointment	

wearers, who have a higher incidence of pseudomonal infection, a topical fluoroquinolone is preferred.

DRY EYE DISEASE

Altered tear-film homeostasis (e.g., altered composition, reduced production, rapid evaporation) and ocular surface inflammation lead to discomfort and blurred vision in patients with dry eye disease. Precipitating factors include poor eyelid function, environmental factors, inflammatory conditions such as Sjögren's syndrome, and use of some ocular or systemic drugs such as antihistamines, retinoids, and selective serotonin reuptake inhibitors (SSRIs). Dry eye disease is most prevalent in females and older adults.[33]

ARTIFICIAL TEARS — Many artificial tear preparations are available; they are usually administered every 4-6 hours, but can be used as often as hourly, depending on symptoms. They usually contain some form of cellulose to lubricate the eye, may contain polyethylene glycol or polyvinyl alcohol to prevent evaporation, and may include a preservative. Preservatives may be irritating and can aggravate ocular surface disease; preservative-free formulations are available. Ophthalmic ointments are usually used at night, but can be used during the day in severe cases. *Lacrisert* is a daily insert that gradually releases hydroxypropylcellulose

Some Available Sizes	Usual Dosage	Cost[1]
3.5 g	0.5 inch q3-4h x 7-10 days	$22.90
3.5 g	0.5 inch q3-4h x 7-10 days	40.30
10 mL	1-2 drops q4h x 7-10 days	51.00
10 mL	1 drop q3h (max 6 doses) x 7-10 days	10.60
10 mL		76.10

after placement into the inferior conjunctival sac; it is FDA-approved for treatment of moderate to severe dry eye syndromes.

TOPICAL CYCLOSPORINE — A 0.05% emulsion of cyclosporine *(Restasis)* is FDA-approved for treatment of dry eye disease.[34] Its mechanism of action is unknown, but is thought to involve immunomodulatory or anti-inflammatory effects. It has been effective in moderate to moderately severe tear dysfunction, producing statistically significant improvement in Schirmer tear test results and other measures of dryness and has been safe, but may take 4-6 weeks to achieve results. Serum cyclosporine concentrations have been undetectable or negligible, and no systemic or topical toxicity has been reported. Transient burning and stinging can occur in the treated eye; addition of topical corticosteroids in the first month may be helpful. A 0.09% cyclosporine solution *(Cequa)* recently FDA-approved for this indication appears to be similar in efficacy, but comparative trials are lacking.[35] Artificial tears available over the counter cost much less than either cyclosporine formulation and should be tried first.

LIFITEGRAST — A 5% ophthalmic solution of lifitegrast *(Xiidra)*, a lymphocyte function-associated antigen-1 (LFA-1) antagonist, is FDA-approved for treatment of dry eye disease. Lifitegrast is thought to reduce

Table 4. Some Prescription Products for Dry Eye Disease			
Drug	**Formulation**	**Usual Adult Dosage**	**Cost[1]**
Cyclosporine ophthalmic emulsion − *Restasis* (Allergan)	0.05% unit-dose vials; multi-dose bottles	1 drop in each eye q12h[2,3]	$557.70
ophthalmic solution − *Cequa* (Sun)	0.09% single-use vials	1 drop in each eye q12h[3]	507.00
Lifitegrast ophthalmic solution − *Xiidra* (Shire)	5% single-use containers	1 drop in each eye q12h[3]	522.20

1. Approximate WAC for 30 days' treatment. WAC = wholesaler acquisition cost or manufacturer's published price to wholesalers; WAC represents a published catalogue or list price and may not represent an actual transactional price. Source: AnalySource® Monthly. November 5, 2019. Reprinted with permission by First Databank, Inc. All rights reserved. ©2019. www.fdbhealth.com/policies/drug-pricing-policy.
2. Before use, the unit-dose vial should be inverted repeatedly until a uniform, white, opaque emulsion forms.
3. Contact lenses should be removed before instillation, but may be replaced 15 minutes after administration.

ocular surface inflammation. It appears to be safe and at least modestly effective, but how it compares to other products remains to be determined.[36]

1. Drugs for allergic disorders. Med Lett Drugs Ther 2017; 59:71.
2. JH Liu et al. Diurnal and nocturnal effects of brimonidine monotherapy on intraocular pressure. Ophthalmology 2010; 117:2075.
3. S Arthur and LB Cantor. Update on the role of alpha-agonists in glaucoma management. Exp Eye Res 2011; 93:271.
4. Two new drugs for glaucoma. Med Lett Drugs Ther 2018; 60:117.
5. R Pujari and HD Jampel. Treating glaucoma with medical marijuana: peering through the smoke. Ophthalmology Glaucoma 2019; 2:201.
6. Cannabis and cannabinoids. Med Lett Drugs Ther 2019; 61:179.
7. X Sun et al. Marijuana for glaucoma: a recipe for disaster or treatment? Yale J Biol Med 2015; 88:265.
8. A Garg and G Gazzard. Selective laser trabeculoplasty: past, present, and future. Eye 2018; 32:863.
9. G Gazzard et al. Selective laser trabeculoplasty versus eye drops for first-line treatment of ocular hypertension and glaucoma (LiGHT): a multicentre randomized controlled trial. Lancet 2019; 393:1505.
10. GM Richter and AL Coleman. Minimally invasive glaucoma surgery: current status and future prospects. Clin Ophthalmol 2016; 10:189.

11. Age-Related Eye Disease Study Research Group. A randomized, placebo-controlled, clinical trial of high-dose supplementation with vitamins C and E, beta carotene, and zinc for age-related macular degeneration and vision loss: AREDS report no. 8. Arch Ophthalmol 2001; 119:1417.

12. Age-Related Eye Disease Study Research Group. Lutein + zeaxanthin and omega-3 fatty acids for age-related macular degeneration: the age-related eye disease study 2 (AREDS2) randomized clinical trial. JAMA 2013; 309:2005.

13. The ATBC Cancer Prevention Study Group. The effect of vitamin E and beta carotene on the incidence of lung cancer and other cancers in male smokers. N Engl J Med 1994; 330:1029.

14. GS Omenn et al. Effects of a combination of beta carotene and vitamin A on lung cancer and cardiovascular disease. N Engl J Med 1996; 334:1150.

15. ER Miller 3rd et al. Meta-analysis: high-dosage vitamin E supplementation may increase all-cause mortality. Ann Intern Med 2005; 142:37.

16. I Bairati et al. Antioxidant vitamins supplementation and mortality: a randomized trial in head and neck cancer patients. Int J Cancer 2006; 119:2221.

17. VEGF inhibitors for AMD and diabetic macular edema. Med Lett Drugs Ther 2015; 57:41.

18. Ranibizumab (Lucentis) for macular degeneration. Med Lett Drugs Ther 2006; 48:85.

19. PJ Rosenfeld et al. Ranibizumab for neovascular age-related macular degeneration. N Engl J Med 2006; 355:1419.

20. BA Frost and MA Kainer. Safe preparation and administration of intravitreal bevacizumab injections. N Engl J Med 2011; 365:2238.

21. CATT Research Group. Ranibizumab and bevacizumab for neovascular age-related macular degeneration. N Engl J Med 2011; 364:1897.

22. U Chakravarthy et al. Alternative treatments to inhibit VEGF in age-related choroidal neovascularization: 2-year findings of the IVAN randomised controlled trial. Lancet 2013; 382:1258.

23. CATT Research Group. Ranibizumab and bevacizumab for treatment of neovascular age-related macular degeneration: two-year results. Ophthalmology 2012; 119:1388.

24. Aflibercept (Eylea) for age-related macular degeneration. Med Lett Drugs Ther 2012; 54:9.

25. PU Dugel et al. HAWK and HARRIER: phase 3, multicenter, randomized, double-masked trials of brolucizumab for neovascular age-related macular degeneration. Ophthalmology 2019 April 12 (epub).

26. Pegaptanib sodium (Macugen) for macular degeneration. Med Lett Drugs Ther 2005; 47:55.

27. SD Solomon et al. Anti-vascular endothelial growth factor for neovascular age-related macular degeneration. Cochrane Database Syst Rev 2014; 3:CD005139.

28. Photodynamic therapy with verteporfin (Visudyne) for macular degeneration. Med Lett Drugs Ther 2000; 42:81.

29. Y Gao et al. Anti-VEGF monotherapy versus photodynamic therapy and anti-VEGF combination treatment for neovascular age-related macular degeneration: a meta-analysis. Invest Ophthalmol Vis Sci 2018; 59:4307.

30. M Teweldemedhin et al. Bacterial profile of ocular infections: a systematic review. BMC Ophthalmol 2017; 17:212.
31. Ophthalmic azithromycin (AzaSite). Med Lett Drugs Ther 2008; 50:11.
32. Ophthalmic besifloxacin (Besivance). Med Lett Drugs Ther 2009; 51:101.
33. EK Akpek et al. Dry eye syndrome preferred practice pattern. Ophthalmology 2019; 126:P286.
34. Ophthalmic cyclosporine (Restasis) for dry eyes. Med Lett Drug Ther 2003; 45:42.
35. Cyclosporine 0.09% solution *(Cequa)* for dry eye disease. Med Lett Drugs Ther 2019; 61:116.
36. Lifitegrast (Xiidra) for dry eye disease. Med Lett Drugs Ther 2016; 58:110.

DRUGS FOR
Gout

Original publication date – March 2019

Drugs for gout reduce the pain and inflammation of acute flares and lower serum urate levels in order to prevent recurrent flares, development of tophi, and joint damage.[1,2]

TREATMENT OF FLARES

NSAIDs — In patients without contraindications to their use (e.g., renal impairment, peptic ulcer disease), acute gout flares can be treated with a nonsteroidal anti-inflammatory drug (NSAID). There is no convincing evidence that indomethacin (*Indocin*, and others), a traditional choice that has a relatively high incidence of adverse effects, is more effective than other NSAIDs, such as ibuprofen (*Motrin*, *Advil*, and others), naproxen (*Naprosyn*, *Aleve*, and others), or COX-2 selective celecoxib (*Celebrex*, and generics). The NSAID should be started as soon as possible after the onset of symptoms and taken regularly (not as needed) until resolution of the flare.

Adverse Effects – All NSAIDs except celecoxib can reversibly inhibit platelet function and prolong bleeding time. Dyspepsia and GI ulceration, perforation, and bleeding can occur with all NSAIDs, often without warning. All NSAIDs inhibit renal prostaglandins, decrease renal blood flow, cause fluid retention, and may cause hypertension and renal failure, particularly in elderly patients. An increased risk of serious cardiovascular events, including myocardial infarction, stroke, and out-of-hospital

Recommendations for Treatment of Gout
▶ Acute flares can be treated with an NSAID, colchicine, or a systemic cortico-steroid. Intra-articular corticosteroid injections can be used if only one or two joints are inflamed.
▶ Urate-lowering drugs should be used to reduce serum urate levels to <6.0 mg/dL, and preferably to <5.0 mg/dL.
▶ When urate-lowering drugs are started, temporary prophylactic use of colchi-cine or an NSAID can prevent paradoxical arthritis flares.
▶ Allopurinol, febuxostat, and probenecid can reduce serum uric acid levels, thereby reducing the frequency of acute flares and the size and number of tophi.
▶ Febuxostat has been associated with a higher risk of cardiovascular death than allopurinol. It should only be used when allopurinol is ineffective or not tolerated.
▶ Pegloticase can be used in patients with severe disease when use of other urate-lowering drugs fails to achieve target serum urate levels or adequate clin-ical improvement.
▶ Loss of excess body weight and avoidance of alcohol have been associated with a reduced risk of gout flares.

cardiac arrest, has been reported with some NSAIDs; the risk appears to be lowest with naproxen. NSAIDs can precipitate asthma symptoms and anaphylactoid reactions in aspirin-sensitive patients. They frequently cause small increases in aminotransferase levels, but serious hepatotoxicity is rare. Cholestatic hepatitis has occurred with celecoxib.

Drug Interactions – NSAIDs can decrease the effectiveness of diuretics, beta blockers, ACE inhibitors, and other antihypertensive drugs. They can increase serum concentrations of lithium and methotrexate, possibly resulting in toxicity. NSAIDs may increase the INR in patients taking warfarin. Patients taking aspirin for cardiovascular protection should not take nonselective NSAIDs regularly because they can interfere with aspirin's antiplatelet effect.

Pregnancy and Lactation – Exposure to NSAIDs during pregnancy or around the time of conception has been associated with an increased risk of miscarriage, but the data are weak. Use of NSAIDs during the third trimester of pregnancy may cause premature closure of the ductus arteriosus and persistent pulmonary hypertension in the neonate, but these effects appear to be uncommon if the drug is stopped 6-8 weeks before delivery.

Data on the safety of NSAID use in breastfeeding women are limited. Secretion of ibuprofen into breast milk is minimal.

COLCHICINE — Colchicine (*Colcrys*, and others) can be used to treat acute flares. It is more likely to be effective if started within 24 hours after symptom onset. Colchicine is also sometimes used for chronic prevention of gout exacerbations.

Adverse Effects – Diarrhea, nausea, and vomiting are common with use of colchicine. Blood dyscrasias have been reported. Neuromyopathy is rare; it typically occurs in elderly patients or in those with hepatic or renal impairment. Overdosage of colchicine can be fatal.

Drug Interactions – Colchicine is a substrate of CYP3A4 and the efflux transporter P-glycoprotein (P-gp); fatalities have been reported rarely in patients taking colchicine with a strong CYP3A4 inhibitor such as clarithromycin (*Biaxin*, and others) or a strong P-gp inhibitor such as cyclosporine (*Neoral*, and others). The dosage of colchicine should be reduced when it is taken concurrently with or within 2 weeks after a CYP3A4 or P-gp inhibitor.[3] Myopathy and rhabdomyolysis have occurred in patients taking colchicine with a statin or a fibrate.

Pregnancy and Lactation – Colchicine has not been adequately studied in pregnant women. In animal studies, it caused embryofetal toxicity and teratogenicity and altered postnatal development. Colchicine is secreted into breast milk.

CORTICOSTEROIDS — Short courses of corticosteroids such as prednisone or methylprednisolone are comparable in efficacy to NSAIDs for treatment of acute flares and may be safer.[4] Intra-articular injection of steroids such as methylprednisolone or triamcinolone is also considered effective and may be useful in patients with one or two inflamed joints.[5]

Table 1. Some Drugs for Gout		
Drug	**Usual Adult Dosage**	**Cost[1]**
Anti-Inflammatory Drugs		
Naproxen – generic _Naprosyn_ (Roche)	Acute: 750 mg PO once, then 250 mg tid Prophylaxis[2,3]: 250 mg PO bid	$7.10 178.00
Ibuprofen – generic	Acute[2]: 800 mg PO tid Prophylaxis[2,3]: 400 mg PO tid	12.20
Colchicine[4] – tablets – generic _Colcrys_ (Takeda) capsules – generic _Mitigare_ (Hikma)	Acute: 1.2 mg PO, then 0.6 mg 1 hour later[5] Prophylaxis[2]: 0.6 mg once/day or bid[5]	 168.40 209.40 156.70 179.50
Prednisone – generic	Acute[3]: 0.5 mg/kg/day PO x 5-10 days	13.00
Anakinra – _Kineret_ (Sobi)	Acute[3]: 100 mg SC once/day x 3 days	658.50
Canakinumab – _Ilaris_ (Novartis)	Acute[3]: 150 mg SC once	16,055.00
Urate-Lowering Drugs		
Allopurinol – generic _Zyloprim_ (Prometheus)	100-900 mg PO daily[6]	12.00 99.10
Febuxostat – generic _Uloric_ (Takeda)	40-80 mg PO once/day[7]	287.50 330.00

1. Approximate wholesale acquisition cost (WAC) for 30 days of prophylactic or urate-lowering treatment at the lowest recommended dosage, for 10 days' treatment of an 80-kg patient with prednisone, or for one course of treatment with anakinra or canakinumab. WAC = wholesaler acquisition cost or manufacturer's published price to wholesalers; WAC represents a published catalogue or list price and may not represent an actual transactional price. Source: AnalySource® Monthly. February 5, 2019. Reprinted with permission by First Databank, Inc. All rights reserved. ©2019. www.fdbhealth.com/policies/drug-pricing-policy.
2. To prevent paradoxical flares during initial urate-lowering therapy; generally continued for 3-6 months after normal serum urate levels are achieved. Colchicine is also sometimes used for chronic prevention of gout flares.
3. Not FDA-approved for this indication.
4. A solution of colchicine 0.6 mg/5 mL (_Gloperba_) has been approved by the FDA for prophylaxis of gout flares in patients initiating urate-lowering therapy.
5. Dosage adjustments may be needed in patients with renal or hepatic impairment and in those taking a CYP3A4 or P-glycoprotein inhibitor.
6. To avoid gout flares, the starting dosage should be ≤100 mg/day. The dose should be increased as needed by 100 mg/day at 2-4 week intervals. Doses >300 mg/day should be divided. The starting dose should be lowered in patients with moderate to severe renal impairment, but should still be titrated up to a maintenance dose that could be higher than 300 mg.
7. In patients with severe renal impairment, the dosage should not exceed 40 mg once daily.

Continued on next page

Table 1. Some Drugs for Gout (continued)		
Drug	**Usual Adult Dosage**	**Cost[1]**
Urate-Lowering Drugs (continued)		
Probenecid – generic	500-1000 mg PO bid	$63.20
Pegloticase – *Krystexxa* (Savient)	8 mg IV q2 weeks	45,845.90[8]
Urate-Lowering/Anti-Inflammatory Drug Combination		
Probenecid/colchicine – generic	500/0.5 mg PO once/day or bid	24.20
8. Cost for 28 days' treatment.		

Adverse Effects – Short-term treatment with a systemic corticosteroid is generally well tolerated, but hyperglycemia, fluid retention, hypertension, and CNS adverse effects can occur. Post-injection flare and septic arthritis can occur after intra-articular corticosteroid injection.

Drug Interactions – Serum concentrations of several systemic corticosteroids (e.g., prednisone, methylprednisolone, triamcinolone) can be decreased with concurrent use of a CYP3A4 inducer and increased with concurrent use of a CYP3A4 inhibitor.[3] Systemic corticosteroids may decrease the effectiveness of antihypertensive and antihyperglycemic drugs.

Pregnancy and Lactation – Low-dose corticosteroids are generally considered safe for short-term use during pregnancy.[6] Glucocorticoids are secreted into breast milk in concentrations lower than in serum.

INTERLEUKIN-1 (IL-1) INHIBITORS — Canakinumab *(Ilaris)*,[7] which is FDA-approved for treatment of systemic juvenile idiopathic arthritis and cryopyrin-associated periodic syndromes (CAPS), has been effective in relieving gout pain and inflammation, but it is expensive.[8] Anakinra *(Kineret)*, which is approved for treatment of rheumatoid arthritis and CAPS, has also reduced the pain and inflammation of gout and is increasingly used off-label for this purpose.[9] These drugs may be options for patients who cannot tolerate or have contraindications to NSAIDs, colchicine, and corticosteroids.

Adverse Effects – Injection-site reactions, infections, neutropenia, thrombocytopenia, and hepatic trans-aminase elevations can occur with use of canakinumab or anakinra.

Drug Interactions – Use of canakinumab or anakinra with TNF inhibitors or other biologics may increase the risk of serious infections and neutropenia and should be avoided.

Pregnancy and Lactation – Canakinumab has not been adequately studied in pregnant women. In animal studies, its use was associated with delays in fetal skeletal development. Monoclonal antibodies are unlikely to cross the placenta in the first trimester but may do so subsequently. Anakinra has not been associated with adverse pregnancy outcomes in small retrospective studies in humans or in animal studies.

There are no data on the presence of canakinumab or anakinra in breast milk or their effects on milk production. Use of anakinra by breastfeeding women has not been associated with adverse effects on breastfed infants, but data are limited.

PREVENTION OF FLARES

Lifestyle changes and urate-lowering drugs should be used to reduce serum urate levels to <6.0 mg/dL, and preferably <5.0 mg/dL; treatment is generally started after resolution of the initial gout flare and continued indefinitely. Asymptomatic, incidental hyperuricemia not associated with gout should not be treated with urate-lowering drugs.

LIFESTYLE CHANGES — Low-purine **diets** have long been recommended for prevention of gout flares, but in a meta-analysis of five studies in 16,760 persons, diet was not found to influence serum urate levels to a clinically significant extent.[10] **Weight loss** in overweight and obese patients with gout has been associated with a reduced risk of acute flares, but data from randomized trials are lacking.[11] In a case-crossover trial in 724 patients with gout, flares were more likely to occur within 24 hours after **alcohol** consumption; the effect was stronger with consumption of larger quantities of alcohol.[12]

PARADOXICAL FLARES — Paradoxical gouty arthritis flares can occur during initiation of urate-lowering therapy. Temporary prophylaxis with colchicine or an NSAID continued for 3-6 months after achieving the target serum urate level can prevent these flares. Colchicine is generally preferred, particularly in older patients, those with comorbidities such as renal impairment or peptic ulcer disease, and those taking anticoagulants or antiplatelet drugs.

XANTHINE OXIDASE INHIBITORS — A xanthine oxidase inhibitor is usually preferred for initial treatment of hyperuricemia. Inhibition of xanthine oxidase blocks conversion of xanthine to uric acid.

Allopurinol (*Zyloprim*, and generics), a xanthine oxidase inhibitor that has been available for many years, reduces the frequency of flares, shrinks tophi, and may prevent urate nephrolithiasis. The dose of allopurinol is titrated, usually from 100 mg/day, until the target urate level is reached. Although a maintenance dose of 300 mg daily is widely used, it often fails to normalize serum urate levels, and doses as high as 900 mg daily may be required. Historical concerns about the safety of allopurinol in patients with renal impairment prompted recommendations for reduced initial and maintenance dosages, but recent data indicate that the drug is safe for use in this population.[13]

Febuxostat *(Uloric*, and generics), a newer xanthine oxidase inhibitor,[14,15] should only be used in patients who have had an inadequate response to or cannot tolerate allopurinol.[16] Use of febuxostat can reduce the frequency of acute gout flares and the size of tophi[17]; its effectiveness in preventing urate nephrolithiasis remains to be established. In patients with severe renal impairment, the dosage of febuxostat should be limited to 40 mg once daily.[18,19]

The FDA has recently required a boxed warning in the febuxostat labeling stating that there is a higher risk of death with febuxostat than with allopurinol. The warning was based on the results of a random-ized, double-blind trial comparing febuxostat to allopurinol in 6190 patients with gout and cardiovascular disease who were followed for a median of 32 months. Cardiovascular death and all-cause mortality occurred more frequently with febuxostat than with allopurinol (CV death 4.3% vs 3.2%, HR 1.34; all-cause mortality 7.8% vs 6.4%, HR 1.22).[16,20] Hyperuricemia itself has been associated with an increased risk of cardiovascular events.[21]

Adverse Effects – Allopurinol can cause cutaneous reactions (including Stevens-Johnson syndrome), hepatic transaminase elevations, leukopenia, and generalized vasculitis. Severe cutaneous reactions are associated with the HLA-B*5801 allele, which is especially common in some Asian popu-lations; patients thought to be at risk should be screened for this allele before taking allopurinol.[22]

Hepatic transaminase elevations can also occur with use of **febuxostat**. Stevens-Johnson syndrome and other hypersensitivity reactions have been reported, but there is no evidence of cross-reactivity with allopurinol.

Drug Interactions – Xanthine oxidase inhibitors can increase the immu-nosuppressive and cytotoxic effects of the purine analogues azathioprine (AZA) and mercaptopurine (6-MP), which are metabolized by xanthine oxidase; coadministration of these drugs with allopurinol or febuxostat should be avoided if possible. Allopurinol can increase serum concen-trations of cyclosporine and prolong the half-life of the sulfonylurea chlorpropamide. It may increase the frequency of skin rash in patients taking ampicillin or amoxicillin. Concurrent use of a thiazide diuretic may increase allopurinol serum concentrations and the risk of toxicity.

Pregnancy and Lactation – Allopurinol and febuxostat have not been associated with an increased risk of abnormal fetal development in animal or human studies, but data in pregnant women are limited.

Allopurinol is secreted into breast milk and its metabolite has been detected in the serum of the breastfed infant.[23] Febuxostat has not been studied in breastfeeding women, but it achieves concentrations in rat milk that are higher than those in serum.

URICOSURIC DRUGS — When a xanthine oxidase inhibitor fails to adequately lower serum urate, adding a uricosuric drug may be beneficial. Patients must have adequate renal function for an optimal response to uricosuric agents.

Probenecid, the only uricosuric drug available in the US, can be used alone or in combination with a xanthine oxidase inhibitor or colchicine for prevention of gout flares. A fixed-dose colchicine/probenecid combination is available.

Lesinurad, a uric acid transporter 1 and organic anion transporter 4 inhibitor that had been available alone *(Zurampic)* and in combination with allopurinol *(Duzallo)*, has been withdrawn from the US market for commercial reasons. A meta-analysis of 5 randomized controlled trials in 1959 patients found that addition of lesinurad to a xanthine oxidase inhibitor did not improve clinical gout-related outcomes such as prevention of flares and resolution of tophi.[24]

Adverse Effects – Probenecid increases the risk of urate nephrolithiasis and is contraindicated in patients with urate nephrolithiasis and in those with high urinary uric acid excretion (>800 mg/day).

Drug Interactions – Probenecid can inhibit tubular secretion of drugs eliminated by organic anion transporters 1 and 3, including methotrexate and many beta-lactam antibiotics. It is contraindicated for use with the NSAID ketorolac. Probenecid can also decrease glucuronidation of acetaminophen and increase formation of the toxic metabolite N-acetyl-p-benzoquinone imine (NAPQI). Salicylates can antagonize the uricosuric effect of probenecid.

Pregnancy and Lactation – Probenecid crosses the placenta and is secreted into breast milk.[25] It is generally considered safe for use during pregnancy.

URICASE — Pegloticase *(Krystexxa)*, an IV pegylated uricase (urate oxidase), converts uric acid to allantoin, an inert water-soluble metabolite cleared by the kidney.[26] Infused every two weeks, pegloticase rapidly lowers serum urate levels in patients with gout.[27] Because of its high cost, potential to cause serious adverse effects, and the need for monitored infusions, pegloticase should be reserved for treatment of highly symptomatic patients and those with severe tophaceous gout in whom other urate-lowering drugs are ineffective or intolerable.

Adverse Effects – Most patients taking pegloticase develop anti-drug antibodies; high titers of these antibodies are associated with reduced drug efficacy and may be responsible for relatively common infusion reactions and a high risk of anaphylaxis (~5%).[28] Lack or loss of urate-lowering response to pegloticase has been considered surrogate evidence for the presence of anti-drug antibodies and an increased risk of serious adverse reactions.[29] Accordingly, serum uric acid levels should be measured before every infusion and discontinuation of pegloticase should be considered if levels exceed 6 mg/dL.

Pegloticase is contraindicated for use in patients with glucose-6-phosphate dehydrogenase (G6PD) deficiency because of the risk of hemolytic anemia and methemoglobinemia; G6PD deficiency should be ruled out before starting therapy.

Drug Interactions – Anti-pegloticase antibodies could theoretically bind to and reduce the efficacy of other pegylated drugs.

Pregnancy and Lactation – Pegloticase has not been adequately studied in pregnant or lactating women. In animal studies, high doses of the drug were associated with decreased fetal and pup body weights.

OTHER DRUGS — The antihypertensive drug **losartan** and the triglyceride-lowering drug **fenofibrate** have uricosuric effects.[30] They may be beneficial for adjunctive prevention of gout flares in patients with other indications for their use.

1. D Khanna et al. 2012 American College of Rheumatology guidelines for management of gout. Part 1: systematic nonpharmacologic and pharmacologic therapeutic approaches to hyperuricemia. Arthritis Care Res (Hoboken) 2012; 64:1431.
2. D Khanna et al. 2012 American College of Rheumatology guidelines for management of gout. Part 2: therapy and antiinflammatory prophylaxis of acute gouty arthritis. Arthritis Care Res (Hoboken) 2012; 64:1447.
3. Inhibitors and inducers of CYP enzymes and P-glycoprotein. Med Lett Drugs Ther 2017 September 18 (epub). Available at: www.medicalletter.org/downloads/CYP_PGP_Tables.pdf.
4. CA Billy et al. Corticosteroid or nonsteroidal antiinflammatory drugs for the treatment of acute gout: A systematic review of randomized controlled trials. J Rheumatol 2018; 45:128.
5. MD Wechalekar et al. Intra-articular glucocorticoids for acute gout. Cochrane Database Syst Rev 2013; 4:CD009920.
6. G Bandoli et al. A review of systemic corticosteroid use in pregnancy and the risk of select pregnancy and birth outcomes. Rheum Dis Clin North Am 2017; 43:489.
7. Canakinumab (Ilaris) for systemic juvenile idiopathic arthritis. Med Lett Drugs Ther 2013; 55:65.
8. N Schlesinger et al. Canakinumab for acute gouty arthritis in patients with limited treatment options: results from two randomised, multicentre, active-controlled, double-blind trials and their initial extensions. Ann Rheum Dis 2012; 71:1839.
9. P Ghosh et al. Treatment of acute gouty arthritis in complex hospitalized patients with anakinra. Arthritis Care Res (Hoboken) 2013; 65:1381.
10. TJ Major et al. Evaluation of the diet wide contribution to serum urate levels: meta-analysis of population based cohorts. BMJ 2018; 363:k3951.
11. SM Nielsen et al. Weight loss for overweight and obese individuals with gout: a systematic review of longitudinal studies. Ann Rheum Dis 2017; 76:1870.
12. T Neogi et al. Alcohol quantity and type on risk of recurrent gout attacks: an internet-based case-crossover study. Am J Med 2014; 127:311.
13. AB Vargas-Santos et al. Association of chronic kidney disease with allopurinol use in gout treatment. JAMA Intern Med 2018; 178:1526.
14. Febuxostat (Uloric) for chronic treatment of gout. Med Lett Drugs Ther 2009; 51:37.
15. MA Becker et al. The urate-lowering efficacy and safety of febuxostat in the treatment of the hyperuricemia of gout: the CONFIRMS trial. Arthritis Res Ther 2010; 12:R63.

16. FDA Drug Safety Communication: FDA adds boxed warning for increased risk of death with gout medicine Uloric (febuxostat). Available at: www.fda.gov/Drugs/DrugSafety/ucm631182.htm. Accessed February 27, 2019.

17. N Dalbeth et al. Lesinurad, a selective uric acid reabsorption inhibitor, in combination with febuxostat in patients with tophaceous gout: findings of a phase III clinical trial. Arthritis Rheumatol 2017; 69:1903.

18. H Yu et al. Safety and efficacy of benzbromarone and febuxostat in hyperuricemia patients with chronic kidney disease: a prospective pilot study. Clin Exp Nephrol 2018 May 14 (epub).

19. KG Saag et al. Efficacy and safety of febuxostat extended and immediate release in patients with gout and renal impairment: a phase III placebo-controlled study. Arthritis Rheumatol 2019; 71:143.

20. WB White et al. Cardiovascular safety of febuxostat or allopurinol in patients with gout. N Engl J Med 2018; 378:1200.

21. ME Kleber et al. Uric acid and cardiovascular events; a Mendelian randomization study. J Am Soc Nephrol 2015; 26:2831.

22. HW Park et al. Efficacy of the HLA-B*58:01 screening test in preventing allopurinol-induced severe cutaneous adverse reactions in patients with chronic renal insufficiency-A prospective study. J Allergy Clin Immunol Pract 2018 Dec 21 (epub).

23. I Kamilli and U Gresser. Allopurinol and oxypurinol in human breast milk. Clin Investig 1993; 71:161.

24. JY Wu et al. Efficacy and safety of lesinurad in patients with hyperuricemia associated with gout: a systematic review and meta-analysis of randomized controlled trials. Pharmacotherapy 2018; 38:1106.

25. KF Ilett et al. Transfer of probenecid and cephalexin into breast milk. Ann Pharmacother 2006; 40:986.

26. Pegloticase (Krystexxa) for treatment of refractory gout. Med Lett Drugs Ther 2011; 53:9.

27. JS Sundy et al. Efficacy and tolerability of pegloticase for the treatment of chronic gout in patients refractory to conventional treatment: two randomized controlled trials. JAMA 2011; 306:711.

28. HS Baraf et al. Infusion-related reactions with pegloticase, a recombinant uricase for the treatment of chronic gout refractory to conventional therapy. J Clin Rheumatol 2014; 20:427.

29. LH Calabrese et al. Frequency, distribution and immunologic nature of infusion reactions in subjects receiving pegloticase for chronic refractory gout. Arthritis Res Ther 2017; 19:191.

30. S Takahashi et al. Effects of combination treatment using anti-hyperuricaemic agents with fenofibrate and/or losartan on uric acid metabolism. Ann Rheum Dis 2003; 62:572.

DRUGS FOR
Chronic Heart Failure

Original publication date – April 2019

Patients with a left ventricular ejection fraction (LVEF) ≤40% are considered to have heart failure with reduced ejection fraction (HFrEF). Patients with a LVEF ≥50% and symptoms of heart failure are considered to have heart failure with preserved ejection fraction (HFpEF). There is little evidence that drug treatment improves clinical outcomes in patients with HFpEF.[1]

All patients with HFrEF should receive one of the drugs that target the renin-angiotensin system (RAS): an angiotensin-converting enzyme (ACE) inhibitor, angiotensin receptor blocker (ARB), or angiotensin receptor-neprilysin inhibitor (ARNI). They should also receive a beta blocker and, if volume overloaded, a diuretic.[2,3]

ACE INHIBITORS — Treatment with an ACE inhibitor improves symptoms (generally over 4-12 weeks), decreases the incidence of hospitalization, and prolongs survival in patients with HFrEF. No data are available showing that any one ACE inhibitor is more effective than any other for treatment of HFrEF. Fosinopril and perindopril have not been approved by the FDA for treatment of heart failure.

Dosage – ACE inhibitors should be started at low doses and titrated to the highest tolerated dose, targeting the usual maximum daily dosages listed in Table 1.

Recommendations for Treatment of HFrEF[1,2]

▶ All patients with HFrEF (LVEF ≤40%), unless contraindicated, should take an angiotensin-converting enzyme (ACE) inhibitor, angiotensin receptor blocker (ARB), or angiotensin receptor-neprilysin inhibitor (ARNI), and a beta blocker.

▶ An ARB is recommended for patients who cannot tolerate an ACE inhibitor because of cough or angioedema.

▶ In patients with NYHA class II-III HFrEF who tolerate an ACE inhibitor or an ARB, replacement with an ARNI is recommended.

▶ In patients who are volume overloaded, a diuretic should be added. Loop diuretics are more effective than thiazide diuretics.

▶ In patients with NYHA class II-IV HFrEF and LVEF ≤35%, a mineralocorticoid receptor antagonist (MRA) should be added.

▶ In black patients with persistently symptomatic NYHA class III-IV HFrEF, a combination of hydralazine and isosorbide dinitrate should be added.

▶ In patients with NYHA class II-III stable chronic HFrEF (LVEF ≤35%) who remain symptomatic in sinus rhythm with a heart rate of ≥70 bpm at rest despite standard therapy including maximally tolerated beta-blocker therapy, addition of ivabradine could be considered.

▶ Digoxin can decrease symptoms and lower the rate of hospitalization for heart failure, but it does not reduce mortality.

1. CW Yancy et al. Circulation 2013; 118:e240.
2. CW Yancy et al. Circulation 2017; 136:e137.

Adverse Effects – The most common adverse effects of ACE inhibitors are related to increased levels of bradykinin (cough and, less commonly, angioedema), suppression of angiotensin II (hypotension and renal insufficiency), and reduction of aldosterone production (hyperkalemia); blood pressure, renal function, and serum potassium concentrations should be monitored. ACE inhibitors should be used cautiously in patients with systolic blood pressure <80 mm Hg, serum creatinine >3 mg/dL, serum potassium >5.0 mEq/L, or bilateral renal artery stenosis. They should not be used in patients with a history of angioedema.[2] Angioedema is more likely to occur in black patients and in women.

Drug Interactions – ACE inhibitors should not be used with an ARB or ARNI. Use of ACE inhibitors with potassium-sparing diuretics, trimethoprim/sulfamethoxazole, or other drugs that increase serum potassium levels increases the risk of hyperkalemia. NSAIDs may decrease the effectiveness of ACE inhibitors and increase the risk of renal impairment. Concurrent use of lithium and an ACE inhibitor can increase lithium serum concentrations; frequent monitoring is recommended. Concurrent use of a thiopurine and an ACE inhibitor can cause leukopenia and anemia. Captopril is a substrate of CYP2D6; use with a CYP2D6 inhibitor may increase its serum concentrations.[4] Quinapril tablets, which contain magnesium, can decrease serum concentrations of oral tetracyclines.[5]

ARBs — Long-term ARB therapy reduces hospitalizations for heart failure and mortality in patients with HFrEF. ARBs can be used in patients who cannot tolerate an ACE inhibitor because of cough or angioedema and in those who were already taking an ARB prior to the diagnosis of heart failure. Candesartan and valsartan are the only ARBs approved by the FDA for treatment of heart failure; losartan has also been widely used.[6,7]

Dosage – ARBs should be started at low doses and titrated to the highest tolerated dose, which is generally achieved by doubling the dose until the usual maximum daily dose (see Table 1) is reached.

Adverse Effects – ARBs, like ACE inhibitors, block the effects of angiotensin II and may cause hypotension, renal insufficiency, and hyperkalemia, but they do not typically cause cough. As with ACE inhibitors, blood pressure, renal function, and serum potassium concentrations should be monitored in patients taking an ARB. Angioedema occurs less often with ARBs than with ACE inhibitors, but it is more likely to occur in patients who had previously developed it while taking an ACE inhibitor.

Drug Interactions – ARBs should not be used with an ACE inhibitor or ARNI. Use of ARBs with potassium-sparing diuretics, trimethoprim/sulfamethoxazole, or other drugs that increase potassium levels increases the risk of hyperkalemia. NSAIDs may decrease the effectiveness of ARBs and increase the risk of renal impairment. Concurrent use of lithium and an ARB can increase lithium serum concentrations; frequent monitoring is recommended. Losartan is a substrate of CYP3A4 and 2C9; inducers

Drugs for Chronic Heart Failure

Table 1. Some Drugs for HFrEF	
Drug	Some Oral Formulations
Angiotensin-Converting Enzyme (ACE) Inhibitors	
Captopril – generic	12.5, 25, 50, 100 mg tabs[3]
Enalapril – generic *Vasotec* (Valeant)	2.5, 5, 10, 20 mg tabs
Fosinopril[4] – generic	10, 20, 40 mg tabs[3]

Lisinopril – generic
  Prinivil (Merck)
  Zestril (Almatica)
	2.5, 5, 10, 20, 40 mg tabs
	5, 10, 20 mg tabs
	2.5, 5, 10, 20, 30, 40 mg tabs

Perindopril[4] – generic	2, 4, 8 mg tabs
Quinapril – generic *Accupril* (Pfizer)	5, 10, 20, 40 mg tabs
Ramipril – generic *Altace* (Pfizer)	1.25, 2.5, 5, 10 mg caps
Trandolapril – generic	1, 2, 4 mg tabs
Angiotensin Receptor Blockers (ARBs)	
Candesartan – generic *Atacand* (AstraZeneca)	4, 8, 16, 32 mg tabs
Losartan[4,5] – generic *Cozaar* (Merck)	25, 50, 100 mg tabs
Valsartan[5] – generic *Diovan* (Novartis)	40, 80, 160, 320 mg tabs[3]
Angiotensin Receptor-Neprilysin Inhibitor	
Sacubitril/valsartan – *Entresto* (Novartis)	24/26, 49/51, 97/103 mg tabs
Beta-Adrenergic Blockers	
Bisoprolol[4] – generic	5, 10 mg tabs[3]

Carvedilol – generic
  Coreg (GSK)
  extended-release – generic
  Coreg CR
	3.125, 6.25, 12.5, 25 mg tabs
	
	10, 20, 40, 80 mg ER caps

ER = extended-release
1. Dosage adjustment may be needed for hepatic or renal impairment.
2. Approximate WAC for 30 days' treatment at the lowest usual maximum adult dosage. WAC = wholesaler acquisition cost or manufacturer's published price to wholesalers; WAC represents a published catalogue or list price and may not represent an actual transactional price. Source: AnalySource® Monthly. March 5, 2019. Reprinted with permission by First Databank, Inc. All rights reserved. ©2019. www.fdbhealth.com/policies/drug-pricing-policy.
3. Available as scored tablets.
4. Not FDA-approved for treatment of heart failure.

Usual Initial Adult Dosage[1]	Usual Maximum Adult Dosage[1]	Cost[2]
6.25 mg tid	50 mg tid	$169.60
2.5 mg bid	20 mg bid	46.30
		1508.90
5-10 mg once/day	40 mg once/day	8.10
2.5-5 mg once/day	40 mg once/day	2.90
		95.40
		398.80
2 mg once/day	16 mg once/day	37.30
5 mg bid	20 mg bid	16.40
		290.60
1.25-2.5 mg once/day	10 mg once/day	13.10
		219.70
1 mg once/day	4 mg once/day	13.80
4-8 mg once/day	32 mg once/day	103.40
		272.20
25-50 mg once/day	150 mg once/day	12.90
		263.10
20-40 mg bid	160 mg bid	36.80
		506.70
49/51 mg bid[6]	97/103 mg bid	509.10
1.25 mg once/day	10 mg once/day	26.30
3.125 mg bid	25 mg bid	4.90
	(50 mg bid for pts >85 kg)	296.50
10 mg once/day	80 mg once/day	205.30
		275.30

5. The FDA has recalled some lots of generic valsartan and losartan products because of the presence of trace amounts of the carcinogens N-nitrosodimethylamine (NDMA), N-nitrosodiethylamine (NDEA), and/or N-nitroso-N-methyl-4-aminobutyric acid (NMBA). In March 2019, the FDA approved a new generic valsartan formulation (Alkem Labs) that does not contain these carcinogens and has temporarily allowed the sale of losartan products that contain NMBA.
6. The initial dosage is 24/26 mg bid for patients currently taking a low-dose ACE inhibitor or ARB or with *de novo* therapy, and for those with an eGFR <30 mL/min/1.73 m², moderate hepatic impairment (Child-Pugh B), or hypotension.

Continued on next page

Drug	Some Oral Formulations
Table 1. Some Drugs for HFrEF (continued)	
Beta-Adrenergic Blockers (continued)	
Metoprolol succinate – generic *Toprol-XL (Aralez)*	25, 50, 100, 200 mg ER tabs[3]
Loop Diuretics	
Bumetanide – generic	0.5, 1, 2 mg tabs
Furosemide – generic *Lasix* (Validus)	20, 40, 80 mg tabs
Torsemide – generic *Demadex* (Meda)	5, 10, 20, 100 mg tabs 10, 20 mg tabs
Mineralocorticoid Receptor Antagonists (MRAs)	
Eplerenone – generic *Inspra* (Pfizer)	25, 50 mg tabs
Spironolactone – generic *Aldactone* (Pfizer)	25, 50, 100 mg tabs[3]
Vasodilators	
Isosorbide dinitrate/hydralazine[9] – *BiDil* (Arbor)[10]	20/37.5 mg tabs
I$_f$ Channel Blocker	
Ivabradine – *Corlanor* (Amgen)	5, 7.5 mg tabs
Digitalis Glycoside	
Digoxin – generic *Digitek* (Mylan) *Digox* (Lannett) *Lanoxin* (Covis)	0.125, 0.25 mg tabs 0.0625, 0.125, 0.1875, 0.25 mg tabs

ER = extended-release
7. Dosage for patients with a serum potassium ≤5 mEq/L and an eGFR ≥50 mL/min/1.73 m², the initial dosage is 25 mg every other day and the maintenance dosage is 25 mg once daily. Dosage adjustments should be made based on serum potassium levels; ≥6.0 mEq/L: withhold dose and restart at 25 mg every other day when levels fall to <5.5 mEq/L; 5.5-5.9 mEq/L: withhold dose if taking 25 mg every other day, reduce dose from 25 mg once daily to 25 mg every other day or from 50 to 25 mg once daily; 5.0-5.4 mEq/L: no adjustment; <5.0 mEq/L: increase dose from 25 mg every other day to 25 mg once daily or from 25 to 50 mg once daily.
8. Dosage for patients with a serum potassium ≤5 mEq/L and an eGFR ≥50 mL/min/1.73 m². For patients with a serum potassium ≤5 mEq/L and an eGFR 30-49 mL/min/1.73 m², the initial dosage is 25 mg every other day. If serum potassium is ≥5.5 mEq/L, withhold dose until levels are <5.0 mEq/L and consider restarting at a reduced dose.

Usual Initial Adult Dosage[1]	Usual Maximum Adult Dosage[1]	Cost[2]
12.5-25 mg once/day	200 mg once/day	$32.20 94.20
0.5-1 mg once/day or bid	10 mg once/day or in divided doses	230.10
20-40 mg once/day or bid	600 mg once/day or in divided doses	31.00 450.90
10-20 mg once/day	200 mg once/day or in divided doses	62.90 962.30
25 mg once/day[7]	50 mg once/day[7]	73.10 342.00
25 mg once/day[8]	50 mg once/day[8]	7.80 133.80
20 mg/37.5 mg tid	40 mg/75 mg tid	610.60
2.5-5 mg bid[11]	7.5 mg bid	442.40
0.125 mg once/day[12] or once every other day	0.125-0.25 mg once/day	36.80 38.00 35.60 372.70

9. Both of these drugs are available generically as single agents. Isosorbide dinitrate is available in 5, 10, 20, and 30-mg tablets and hydralazine in 10, 25, 50, and 100-mg tablets.
10. FDA-approved as adjunctive therapy for treatment of heart failure in black patients.
11. An initial dosage of 2.5 mg bid can be used in patients with underlying conduction disease or those at higher risk of hemodynamic compromise.
12. Usual initial dosage is 0.125 mg every other day in patients with CrCl <30 mL/min.

of these isozymes could decrease its efficacy and inhibitors could increase its serum concentrations and toxicity.[4] Valsartan is a substrate of organic anion transporting polypeptide (OATP) 1B1; concomitant use with drugs that inhibit OATP1B1, such as atorvastatin (*Lipitor*, and others), could increase valsartan serum concentrations.[8]

ARNI – A combination of the ARB valsartan and the neprilysin inhibitor sacubitril *(Entresto)* is FDA-approved to reduce the risk of hospitalization for heart failure and cardiovascular death in patients with HFrEF.[9] The inhibition of neprilysin, which degrades several vasoactive peptides, enhances vasodilation and sodium excretion.

In a randomized clinical trial in patients with HFrEF (PARADIGM-HF), the combination of sacubitril and a standard dose of valsartan (160 mg twice daily) was significantly more effective than a dose of the ACE inhibitor enalapril (10 mg twice daily) in reducing the rate of death from cardiovascular causes or hospitalization for heart failure (21.8% vs 26.5%).[10,11] A study comparing sacubitril/valsartan with valsartan alone is in progress.

To further reduce morbidity and mortality in patients with chronic symptomatic New York Heart Association (NYHA) class II–III HFrEF who are tolerating an ACE inhibitor or an ARB, ACC/AHA/HFSA guidelines now recommend replacement with an ARNI.[3] Because a relatively low dose of enalapril was used in the PARADIGM-HF trial, some clinicians recommend reserving sacubitril/valsartan for patients who remain symptomatic on optimal doses of an ACE inhibitor or an ARB.

Dosage – Patients previously taking a moderate- to high-dose ACE inhibitor or ARB can be started on sacubitril/valsartan 49/51 mg twice daily. Low-dose sacubitril/valsartan (24/26 mg twice daily) is recommended for patients currently taking a low-dose ACE inhibitor or ARB or with *de novo* therapy, and for those with an eGFR <30 mL/min/1.73 m^2, moderate hepatic impairment (Child-Pugh B), or hypotension. The dose should be doubled every 2 weeks to a target of 97/103 mg twice daily as tolerated.

Adverse Effects – Hypotension, renal insufficiency, and hyperkalemia can occur. As with ACE inhibitors and ARBs, blood pressure, renal function, and serum potassium concentrations should be monitored in patients taking an ARNI. Angioedema occurs less often with sacubitril/valsartan than with ACE inhibitors, but neprilysin inhibition can cause angioedema; patients with a history of angioedema should not take an ARNI.[3]

Drug Interactions – *Entresto* is contraindicated for use with or within 36 hours after the last dose of an ACE inhibitor because of the risk of angioedema. It also should not be used with an ARB. Concurrent use of sacubitril/valsartan and potassium-sparing diuretics, trimethoprim/sulfamethoxazole, or other drugs that increase potassium levels increases the risk of hyperkalemia. Worsening of renal function and acute renal failure could occur in patients taking sacubitril/valsartan and NSAIDs concurrently. Concurrent use of lithium with an ARB can increase lithium serum concentrations; frequent monitoring is recommended. Valsartan is a substrate of OATP1B1; concomitant use with drugs that inhibit OATP1B1, such as atorvastatin, could increase valsartan serum concentrations.[4,8]

BETA BLOCKERS — Long-term therapy with a beta blocker improves symptoms and clinical outcomes in patients with HFrEF. Carvedilol, metoprolol succinate, and bisoprolol have been shown to reduce the rates of hospitalization and death in patients with HFrEF. Bisoprolol is not approved by the FDA for treatment of heart failure.

Dosage – Beta blockers should be started at low doses and increased gradually, usually at 2-week intervals, to the highest tolerated dose. Full clinical benefits may not occur for 3-6 months or longer, and transient worsening of symptoms can occur following dose increases.

Adverse Effects – Fatigue, hypotension, bradycardia, asymptomatic fluid retention, and worsening heart failure may occur during the first few weeks of treatment. Increasing the dose of a concurrent diuretic may be helpful. Carvedilol, which has vasodilatory activity, may cause more hypotension than metoprolol or bisoprolol. Beta blockers should be used cautiously, if at all, in patients with severe bradycardia or significant asthma; metoprolol and bisoprolol may have a lower risk of broncho-spasm because of their beta-1 selectivity.

Drug Interactions – Carvedilol and metoprolol are substrates of CYP2D6; concurrent use with a CYP2D6 inhibitor may increase their serum concentrations and their toxicity. Carvedilol is also an inhibitor of the drug transporter P-glycoprotein (P-gp) and can increase serum concentrations of P-gp substrates such as digoxin. Bisoprolol is a substrate of CYP3A4; use with CYP3A4 inducers may decrease its efficacy.[4,5]

DIURETICS — Most patients with heart failure have fluid retention. Diuretics relieve symptoms in such patients, but their effect on survival is unclear. Diuretics provide symptomatic relief of pulmonary and periph-eral edema more rapidly than other drugs used for the treatment of heart failure. Loop diuretics such as furosemide, bumetanide, or torsemide are more effective in patients with heart failure than thiazide-type diuretics such as hydrochlorothiazide or chlorthalidone. Torsemide and bumeta-nide are better absorbed than furosemide, but there is no clinical evidence that either is more effective than furosemide.

Dosage – Diuretics should be started at a low dose, which can be titrated upward until urine output increases and weight decreases. Higher starting doses can be used in patients with renal impairment or prior refractoriness to loop diuretics. Intravenous administration, concurrent use of 2 diuretics (a loop and a thiazide-like diuretic), or addition of a mineralocorticoid receptor antagonist (MRA) can sometimes overcome diuretic resistance.

Adverse Effects – The most common adverse effect of loop diuretics is hypokalemia. Diuretics can also cause worsening of renal function.

Drug Interactions – NSAIDs can decrease the effectiveness of diuretics. Concurrent use of lithium and a diuretic could increase lithium serum concentrations; frequent monitoring is recommended. Torsemide is a substrate of CYP2C9; use with inducers of CYP2C9 could decrease its efficacy and use with 2C9 inhibitors could increase serum concentrations and its toxicity.[4,5]

MRAs — When added to standard therapy in patients with HFrEF, mineralocorticoid receptor antagonists (MRAs) have been shown to reduce the risk of hospitalization and death.[12,13] Addition of eplerenone or spironolactone is recommended for patients with NYHA class II-IV heart failure with a LVEF ≤35%. Eplerenone is similar in effectiveness to spironolactone and has less anti-androgenic activity, but it costs more.

Dosage – Initial dosage and dose adjustments of MRAs are based on serum potassium levels (see Table 1).

Adverse Effects – Hyperkalemia occurs frequently with MRAs; the risk is higher in patients also taking an ACE inhibitor or an ARB, and in those with renal impairment. MRAs should not be used in patients with serum potassium >5.0 mEq/L and in those with reduced renal function (baseline serum creatinine >2.0 mg/dL for women or >2.5 mg/dL for men, or an eGFR <30 mL/min/1.73 m^2). Renal function and potassium and serum creatinine concentrations should be monitored during treatment. Spironolactone has anti-androgenic activity and can cause erectile dysfunction and painful gynecomastia in men, menstrual irregularities in women, and hair loss in both men and women; the incidence of these effects is lower with eplerenone.

Drug Interactions – Use of an MRA with other drugs that increase serum potassium levels increases the risk of hyperkalemia. Eplerenone is a CYP3A4 substrate; use with CYP3A4 inducers could decrease its serum concentrations and efficacy and use with 3A4 inhibitors could increase its serum concentrations and toxicity.[4,5]

VASODILATORS — In black patients with heart failure who remain symptomatic on standard therapy, the addition of a fixed-dose combination of isosorbide dinitrate and hydralazine *(BiDil)* significantly reduces symptoms, first hospitalization for heart failure, and mortality.[14] Its benefit in non-black patients is less well established, but its use can be considered in those who cannot tolerate an ACE inhibitor or an ARB.

Dosage – Isosorbide dinitrate/hydralazine should be started at a low dose, which can be titrated upward every 2-4 weeks (see Table 1). Patients should be monitored for hypotension.

Adverse Effects – Isosorbide dinitrate/hydralazine can cause hypotension, headache, and dizziness. Hydralazine alone can cause tachycardia, peripheral neuritis, and a lupus-like syndrome.

Drug Interactions – Phosphodiesterase 5 (PDE5)inhibitors, such as sildenafil (*Viagra, Revatio,* and generics), should not be taken concurrently with isosorbide dinitrate/hydralazine because of the risk of additive hypotensive effects.

IVABRADINE — The I_f channel inhibitor ivabradine *(Corlanor)* slows heart rate in patients in sinus rhythm by inhibiting the cardiac pacemaker I_f current. It has no effect on contractility. In a randomized trial in patients with symptomatic heart failure, LVEF ≤35%, and a resting heart rate >70 bpm despite beta blocker therapy, addition of ivabradine significantly reduced the rates of hospitalization for worsening heart failure and death due to heart failure, but not cardiovascular death, compared to placebo. However, these patients did not receive maximally-tolerated beta-blocker therapy. They were taking low doses of beta blockers; only 26% were at the target dose and only 56% were at 50% of the target dose.[15,16]

Dosage – The initial dosage of ivabradine is 5 mg twice daily with meals. A lower starting dosage of 2.5 mg twice daily can be used in patients with underlying conduction disease or those at higher risk of hemodynamic compromise. The dose should be adjusted every two weeks to a maximum of 7.5 mg twice daily.

Adverse Effects – Symptomatic bradycardia, hypertension, atrial fibrillation, and visual effects (transient increases in brightness due to inhibition of electric currents in the retina) have been reported with ivabradine. It should not be used in patients with atrial fibrillation.

Drug Interactions – Ivabradine is a substrate of CYP3A4; use with strong CYP3A4 inhibitors is contraindicated and use with 3A4 inducers or moderate 3A4 inhibitors should be avoided.[4,5]

DIGOXIN — In patients with HFrEF, digoxin can decrease heart failure symptoms, increase exercise tolerance, and decrease hospitalization rates, but it does not prolong survival. A low dose (0.125 mg daily) is sometimes used in patients with HFrEF that has not responded to standard therapy; digoxin levels of 0.5-0.9 ng/mL are recommended. Dose adjustments based on renal function, age, and concomitant medications may be required. The most common adverse effects of digoxin are conduction disturbances, cardiac arrhythmias, nausea, vomiting, confusion, and visual disturbances.

PREGNANCY — **ACE inhibitors**, **ARBs**, and the **ARNI** are contraindicated for use during pregnancy because they increase the risk of fetal renal failure and death. **Beta blockers** have been associated with fetal growth restriction, but beta-1-selective drugs (e.g., metoprolol) are less likely to cause this effect. A review of 13 population-based studies found that use of beta blockers in the first trimester was not associated with an overall increase in congenital malformations, but in some studies, their use has been associated with increased rates of cleft lip/palate and cardiovascular and neural tube defects.[17] **Diuretic therapy** should be initiated with caution during pregnancy because volume depletion caused by these drugs in their first weeks of use may reduce uteroplacental perfusion; women already taking a diuretic who become pregnant can generally continue taking it. **MRAs** are teratogenic and should not be used during pregnancy. No data are available on the safety of **isosorbide dinitrate/ hydralazine** for use during pregnancy. Fetal toxicity and cardiac teratogenic effects have occurred in animal studies with **ivabradine**; women of childbearing age should use effective contraception while taking the drug. Pregnant women taking ivabradine should be monitored for bradycardia, destabilization of heart failure, and preterm birth (in the third trimester). **Digoxin** is generally considered safe for use during pregnancy.

LACTATION — Some **ACE inhibitors**, including captopril, enalapril, perindopril, and quinapril, have been studied in lactating women, and although low levels of these drugs have been found in breast milk, no adverse effects are expected in breastfed infants. There are no data on the presence of **ARBs** or the **ARNI** in breast milk. **Metoprolol** is the beta blocker of choice for treatment of heart failure in breastfeeding women; beta blockers with low protein binding (e.g., **bisoprolol**) are more likely to be excreted into breast milk and should be avoided. Decreased fluid volume caused by **diuretics** may impact lactation; diuretics have been used to intentionally suppress lactation. There are no data on the presence of loop diuretics in breast milk. Thiazide diuretics are present in breast milk in low concentrations; no adverse effects are expected in breastfed infants. **Spironolactone** appears to be safe for use in breastfeeding women. There are no data on the presence of **eplerenone** or **isosorbide dinitrate/hydralazine** in breast milk. Breastfeeding should be avoided in women taking **ivabradine**. **Digoxin** levels in breast milk are low; avoidance of breastfeeding for 2 hours post-dose is recommended.

1. P Rossignol et al. Heart failure drug treatment. Lancet 2019; 393:1034.
2. CW Yancy et al. 2013 ACCF/AHA guideline for the management of heart failure: a report of the American College of Cardiology Foundation/American Heart Association Task Force on practice guidelines. Circulation 2013; 128:e240.
3. CW Yancy et al. 2017 ACC/AHA/HFSA focused update of the 2013 ACCF/AHA guideline for the management of heart failure: a report of the American College of Cardiology/American Heart Association Task Force on Clinical Practice Guidelines and the Heart Failure Society of America. Circulation 2017; 136:e137.
4. Inhibitors and inducers of CYP enzymes and P-glycoprotein. Med Lett Drugs Ther 2017; September 18 (epub). Available at: www.medicalletter.org/downloads/CYP_PGP_Tables.pdf.
5. Drug Interactions from The Medical Letter. Available at: www.medicalletter.org/subDIO.
6. H Svanström et al. Association of treatment with losartan vs candesartan and mortality among patients with heart failure. JAMA 2012; 307:1506.
7. MA Konstam et al. Effects of high-dose versus low-dose losartan on clinical outcomes in patients with heart failure (HEAAL study): a randomised, double-blind trial. Lancet 2009; 374:1840.
8. FDA. Drug development and drug interactions: table of substrates, inhibitors and inducers. Available at www.fda.gov. Accessed March 27, 2019.

9. Sacubitril/valsartan (Entresto) for heart failure. Med Lett Drugs Ther 2015; 57:107.
10. JJ McMurray et al. Angiotensin-neprilysin versus enalapril in heart failure. N Engl J Med 2014; 371:993.
11. O Vardeny et al. Combined neprilysin and renin-angiotensin system inhibition for the treatment of heart failure. JACC Heart Fail 2014; 2:663.
12. F Zannad et al. Eplerenone in patients with systolic heart failure and mild symptoms. N Engl J Med 2011; 364:11.
13. B Pitt et al. The effect of spironolactone on morbidity and mortality in patients with severe heart failure. Randomized Aldactone Evaluation Study Investigators. N Engl J Med 1999; 341:709.
14. AL Taylor et al. Combination of isosorbide dinitrate and hydralazine in blacks with heart failure. New Engl J Med 2004; 351:2049.
15. K Swedberg et al. Ivabradine and outcomes in chronic heart failure (SHIFT): a randomised placebo-controlled study. Lancet 2010; 376:875.
16. Ivabradine (Corlanor) for heart failure. Med Lett Drugs Ther 2015; 57:75.
17. MY Yacoob et al. The risk of congenital malformations associated with exposure to β-blockers early in pregnancy: a meta-analysis. Hypertension 2013; 62:375.

Insect Repellents

Original publication date – August 2019

Use of insect repellents is strongly recommended by the Centers for Disease Control and Prevention (CDC) and the Environmental Protection Agency (EPA) to prevent infections transmitted by mosquitoes and ticks. Insect repellents applied to exposed skin should be used in conjunction with other preventive measures such as wearing pants and long-sleeved shirts, and avoiding outdoor activities during peak mosquito-biting times.[1] Mosquitoes can transmit Zika, chikungunya, dengue, West Nile, eastern equine encephalitis, and yellow fever viruses, as well as malaria. Ticks can transmit Lyme disease, rickettsial diseases such as Rocky Mountain spotted fever, and viruses such as Powassan virus.

DEET — The topical insect repellent N,N-diethyl-*m*-toluamide (DEET) is highly effective against mosquito and tick bites.[2] It also repels chiggers, fleas, gnats, and some flies. DEET is available in concentrations of 5-99%; higher concentrations typically provide longer-lasting protection,[3] but increasing the concentration above 50% has not been shown to improve efficacy. Long-acting polymer-based or liposomal DEET formulations containing concentrations of 30-34% have been shown to protect against mosquitoes for up to 12 hours. The CDC recommends using concentrations ≥20% in adults for protection against both mosquitoes and ticks.

Reviews of the safety and toxicity of topically applied DEET indicate that it is generally safe.[2,4] Toxic and allergic reactions to DEET have

Summary: Insect Repellents

▸ DEET is highly effective against mosquito and tick bites and is generally safe.
▸ Picaridin appears to be as effective against mosquitoes as equivalent concentrations of DEET and may be better tolerated on the skin. It also repels ticks.
▸ IR3535 at concentrations ≥10% and oil of lemon eucalyptus (OLE) can also be effective in repelling mosquitoes and ticks.
▸ Published data on the efficacy of 2-undecanone are limited.
▸ Citronella oil-based insect repellents provide short-term protection against mosquitoes, but not ticks. Other essential oils provide limited and variable protection against mosquitoes.
▸ Wearing clothing treated with the insecticide permethrin in addition to using DEET or picaridin on exposed skin may provide the best protection against mosquitoes and ticks.
▸ Wearable devices such as wristbands are not effective.

been uncommon, and serious adverse effects are rare.[4] Rashes ranging from mild irritation to urticaria and bullous eruptions have been reported. Patients find that some DEET formulations feel uncomfortably oily or sticky on their skin. DEET can damage clothing made from synthetic fibers and plastics on eyeglass frames and watches.

Children – The American Academy of Pediatrics recommends using DEET formulations containing concentrations of 10-30% on children and infants >2 months old. Neurologic adverse events have occurred in infants and children, usually with prolonged or excessive use that sometimes included ingestion of the product.

PICARIDIN — Picaridin provides protection against mosquitoes, ticks, flies, fleas, and chiggers. It is available in concentrations of 5-20%; higher concentrations typically provide longer lasting protection.[5] Picaridin appears to be at least as effective against mosquitoes as DEET at similar concentrations.[6]

Picaridin can cause skin and eye irritation, but it appears to be better tolerated on the skin than DEET. It is odorless, non-greasy, and does not damage fabric or plastic, but it can discolor leather and vinyl. In a review of data from US poison centers, ingestion of picaridin-based insect repellents resulted in only minor toxicity (mild oral or skin irritation, mild GI symptoms) that did not require referral to a healthcare facility.[7]

Children – The American Academy of Pediatrics recommends formulations of picaridin containing concentrations of 5-10% for use on children as an alternative to DEET.

IR3535 — IR3535 (3-[N-Butyl-N-acetyl]-amino-propionic acid, ethyl ester), a synthetic version of β-alanine, repels mosquitoes, deer ticks, and flies. It is available in concentrations of 7.5% and 20% in the US (see Table 1). Concentrations ≥10% have been found to be effective against mosquito bites for several hours.[8] Two studies found the 7.5% concentration to be ineffective.[3,9] IR3535 can cause eye irritation, and it may damage clothing and plastics.

Children – According to the EPA, IR3535 is safe for use on children >2 months old.

OIL OF LEMON EUCALYPTUS — Oil of lemon eucalyptus (OLE; *p*-menthane-3,8-diol [PMD]), which repels mosquitoes, ticks, flies, gnats, and biting midges, occurs naturally in the lemon eucalyptus plant.[2] It is chemically synthesized for commercial use as a repellent. In field studies against malaria-transmitting mosquitoes, OLE provided up to 6 hours of protection against mosquito bites.[8] It has demonstrated efficacy equivalent to that of DEET against mosquitoes in some laboratory and field studies.[10] OLE can cause eye and skin irritation, including allergic skin reactions.[11]

Children – OLE products are not recommended for use on children <3 years old.

2-UNDECANONE — A relatively new insect repellent, 2-undecanone is derived from the wild tomato plant.[12] A synthetic version is commercially

Table 1. Some Insect Repellents

Repellent	Formulation
DEET (N,N-diethyl-*m*-toluamide)	
Cutter All Family Mosquito Wipes	7.15% wipes
Off! Family Care	15% aerosol spray
Off! Deep Woods VII	25% pump spray
Sawyer Family Controlled Release	20% lotion
Ultrathon[2]	34% lotion
Repel 100	98.11% pump spray[3]
Picaridin	
Cutter Advanced	5.75% wipes
Avon Skin So Soft Bug Guard Plus Picaridin	10% aerosol spray
Natrapel 8 hour	20% pump spray
Sawyer Picaridin Lotion	20% lotion
IR3535 (3-[N-acetyl-N-butyl]-aminopropionic acid, ethyl ester)	
Avon Skin So Soft Bug Guard Plus IR3535[4]	7.5% lotion
Coleman Skin Smart	20% aerosol spray
Oil of Lemon Eucalyptus (OLE; *p*-menthane-3,8-diol [PMD])[5]	
Off! Botanicals	10% pump spray
Coleman Botanicals	30% pump spray
Repel Lemon Eucalyptus	30% pump spray
2-undecanone	
HOMS Bite Blocker BioUD Insect Repellent and Clothing Treatment	7.75% pump spray
Citronella[6]	
Buzz Away Extreme	1.0% pump spray[7]

1. Approximate duration of protection against mosquitoes for repellents applied to exposed skin, according to protection times approved by the EPA for product labels; for most products, the duration of protection against ticks is expected to be similar (except 2-undecanone, which repels ticks for 2 hours). Products listed in this database are those with an EPA registration number, which indicates the company provided the EPA with technical information on the safety of the product and its effectiveness against mosquitoes and/or ticks. Although this technical information is based on scientific testing guidelines and approved study methods, there are variations in the resulting protection times because of differences in testing conditions. Duration of protection may be affected by ambient temperature, activity level, amount of perspiration, exposure to water, and other factors. Available at: www.epa.gov/insect-repellents/find-insect-repellent-right-you. Accessed August 15, 2019.

Duration of Protection[1]	Comments
2 hrs 6 hrs 8 hrs 11 hrs 12 hrs 10 hrs	Highly effective broad-spectrum repellent; safe on pregnant women and children >2 months old; may feel oily on the skin
8 hrs 6 hrs 8 hrs 14 hrs	Appears to be as effective against mosquitoes as similar concentrations of DEET; also repels ticks; safe on pregnant women and children >2 months old; odorless, non-greasy
2 hrs 8 hrs	Concentrations ≥10% effective against mosquitoes; also repels ticks; safe on pregnant women and children >2 months old
2 hrs 6 hrs 6 hrs	Effective for repelling mosquitoes and ticks; avoid on children <3 years old; safe on pregnant women
5 hrs	Limited data available; may have strong odor
2 hrs	Short-term effectiveness against mosquitoes; probably not effective against ticks

2. Long-acting polymer-based formulation developed for the US military.
3. There is no evidence that concentrations of DEET above 50% are more effective.
4. Contains IR3535 combined with sunscreen; products that contain both an insect repellent and a sunscreen are not recommended because the sunscreen may need to be reapplied more often and in greater amounts than the repellent.
5. Oil of lemon eucalyptus (OLE) is not the same as pure, essential oil of lemon eucalyptus, which is not recommended for use as an insect repellent.
6. Citronella is also available in a variety of brand name products that are not EPA registered.
7. Also contains castor oil (8%), geranium oil (6%), soybean oil (3%), peppermint oil (0.5%), and lemon-grass oil (0.25%).

Continued on next page

Table 1. Some Insect Repellents (continued)	
Repellent	**Formulation**
Permethrin	
Sawyer Premium Permethrin Clothing	0.5% pump spray
Repel Permethrin Clothing and Gear	0.5% aerosol spray

available in a 7.75% spray formulation *(BioUD)*. Published data on the efficacy of 2-undecanone are limited.[2] According to the product label, *BioUD* is effective for up to 4.5 hours against mosquitoes and up to 2 hours against ticks. It can have a strong odor.

CITRONELLA — Citronella oil-based insect repellents provide short-term protection against mosquitoes, but they are probably not effective against ticks. In laboratory studies, various concentrations of citronella oil were less effective than DEET against mosquito bites in duration of protection.[13] The protection times for most citronella oil products are 2 hours or less, and they can cause skin irritation.

OTHER ESSENTIAL OILS — Essential oils obtained from raw botanical material, including clove, geraniol, catnip, and patchouli, provide limited and variable protection against mosquitoes. High concentrations can be irritating to the skin.[14,15]

SUNSCREENS AND INSECT REPELLENTS — Topical insect repellents can be used with sunscreens; the repellent should be applied after the sunscreen. Applying DEET after sunscreen has been shown to reduce the sun protection factor (SPF) of the sunscreen, but applying sunscreen after DEET may increase absorption of DEET. The CDC does not recommend use of products that combine a sunscreen with an insect repellent because the sunscreen may need to be reapplied more often and in greater amounts than the repellent.

Duration of Protection[1]	Comments
– –	For use on clothing and gear; avoid on exposed skin; effective against mosquitoes and ticks

PERMETHRIN — A synthetic pyrethroid contact insecticide, permethrin can be sprayed on clothing, mosquito nets, tents, and sleeping bags to repel and kill mosquitoes and ticks. Permethrin-impregnated clothing is available commercially; it remains active for several weeks through multiple launderings with minimal transfer to the skin.[16] An indoor laboratory study found that subjects wearing permethrin-treated sneakers and socks were 73.6 times less likely to be bitten by a tick than those wearing untreated footwear.[17] Studies in outdoor workers in North Carolina wearing uniforms treated with a long-lasting formulation of permethrin using a commercially available factory-based method found that the clothing protected against mosquito and tick bites for at least 1 year.[18,19] No significant adverse effects have been reported from wearing permethrin-treated clothing.[11]

WEARABLE DEVICES — Several insect repellents, including DEET, OLE, and citronella, are commercially available in wearable devices such as wristbands. These devices are not effective.[20,21]

PREGNANCY — The CDC considers EPA-registered formulations of DEET, picaridin, IR3535, OLE, and 2-undecanone safe for use during pregnancy.[22] According to the EPA, there is no evidence that exposure to permethrin results in adverse effects in pregnant or nursing women or developmental adverse effects in their children.[23] In its Zika virus prevention guidelines, the American College of Obstetricians and Gynecologists recommended that pregnant women traveling to areas where Zika has been reported use an EPA-registered DEET product and permethrin-treated clothing, cover exposed skin, and stay in air-conditioned or indoor areas.[24,25]

1. CDC/EPA. Joint statement on insect repellents from the Environmental Protection Agency and the Centers for Disease Control and Prevention. July 17, 2014. Available at: www.epa.gov. Accessed August 15, 2019.
2. QD Nguyen et al. Insect repellents: an updated review for the clinician. J Am Acad Dermatol 2018 Nov 2 (epub).
3. MS Fradin and JF Day. Comparative efficacy of insect repellents against mosquito bites. N Engl J Med 2002; 347:13.
4. Chen-Hussey et al. Assessment of methods used to determine the safety of the topical insect repellent N,N-diethyl-*m*-toluamide (DEET). Parasit Vectors 2014; 7:173.
5. Picaridin – a new insect repellent. Med Lett Drugs Ther 2005; 47:46.
6. L Goodyer and S Schofield. Mosquito repellents for the traveller: does picaridin provide longer protection than DEET? J Travel Med 2018; 25(suppl_1):S10.
7. NP Charlton et al. The toxicity of picaridin containing insect repellent reported to the National Poison Data System. Clin Toxicol (Phila) 2016; 54:655.
8. LI Goodyer et al. Expert review of the evidence base for arthropod bite avoidance. J Travel Med 2010; 17:182.
9. SP Frances et al. Comparative field evaluation of repellent formulations containing DEET and IR3535 against mosquitoes in Queensland, Australia. J Am Mosq Control Assoc 2009; 25:511.
10. SP Carroll and J Loye. PMD, a registered botanical mosquito repellent with DEET-like efficacy. J Am Mosq Control Assoc 2006; 22:507.
11. JH Diaz. Chemical and plant-based insect repellents: efficacy, safety, and toxicity. Wilderness Environ Med 2016; 27:153.
12. BE Witting-Bissinger et al. Novel arthropod repellent, BioUD, is an efficacious alternative to DEET. J Med Entomol 2008; 45:891.
13. C Kongkaew et al. Effectiveness of citronella preparations in preventing mosquito bites: systematic review of controlled laboratory experimental studies. Trop Med Int Health 2011; 16:802.
14. Y Trongtokit et al. Comparative repellency of 38 essential oils against mosquito bites. Phytother Res 2005; 19:303.
15. MY Lee. Essential oils as repellents against arthropods. Biomed Res Int. 2018 Oct 2 (epub).
16. KM Sullivan et al. Bioabsorption and effectiveness of long-lasting permethrin-treated uniforms over three months among North Carolina outdoor workers. Parasit Vector 2019; 12:52.
17. NJ Miller et al. Tick bite protection with permethrin-treated summer-weight clothing. J Med Entomol 2011; 48:327.
18. MF Vaughn et al. Long-lasting permethrin impregnateduniforms: a randomized-controlled trial for tick bite prevention. Am J Prev Med 2014; 46:473.
19. B Londono-Renteria et al. Long-lasting permethrin-impregnated clothing protects against mosquito bites in outdoor workers. Am J Trop Med Hyg 2015; 93:869.

20. SD Rodriguez et al. Efficacy of some wearable devices compared with spray-on insect repellents for the yellow fever mosquito, *Aedes aegypti* (L.) *(Diptera: Culcidae)*. J Insect Sci 2017; 17:24.

21. RV Patel et al. EPA-registered repellents for mosquitoes transmitting emerging viral disease. Pharmacotherapy 2016; 36:1272.

22. CDC. Zika virus. Prevent mosquito bites. Available at www.cdc.gov/zika/prevention/prevent-mosquito-bites.html. Accessed August 15, 2019.

23. US Environmental Protection Agency. Repellent-treated clothing. Last updated March 29, 2016. Available at: www.epa.gov/insect-repellents/repellent-treated-clothing. Accessed August 15, 2019.

24. American College of Obstetricians and Gynecologists. Practice advisory interim guidance for care of obstetric patients during a Zika virus outbreak. Available at www.acog.org/Clinical-Guidance-and-Publications/Practice-Advisories/Practice-Advisory-Interim-Guidance-for-Care-of-Obstetric-Patients-During-a-Zika-Virus-Outbreak#prevention. Accessed August 15, 2019.

25. BJ Wylie et al. Insect repellants during pregnancy in the era of the Zika virus. Obstet Gynecol 2016; 128:1111.

Lipid-Lowering Drugs

Original publication date – February 2019

Cholesterol management guidelines from the American College of Cardiology/American Heart Association Task Force have recently been published.[1] See Table 1 for a brief summary of their recommendations.

STATINS — HMG-CoA reductase inhibitors (statins) remain the drugs of choice for most patients who require lipid-lowering therapy. Statins block the rate-limiting step in cholesterol synthesis. The subsequent reduction in hepatic cholesterol causes upregulation of low-density lipoprotein (LDL) receptors, increasing uptake and clearance of LDL-cholesterol (LDL-C) from the blood. High-intensity statin therapy (atorvastatin 40-80 mg/day, rosuvastatin 20-40 mg/day) reduces LDL-C levels by ≥50%, moderate-intensity statin therapy (e.g., atorvastatin 10-20 mg/day, rosuvastatin 5-10 mg/day, simvastatin 20-40 mg/day) reduces LDL-C levels by 30-49%, and low-intensity statin therapy (e.g., pravastatin 10-20 mg/day, lovastatin 20 mg/day) reduces LDL-C levels by <30%. Statins also decrease very low-density lipoprotein cholesterol (VLDL-C) and triglyceride levels and modestly increase high-density lipoprotein cholesterol (HDL-C) levels.

Primary Prevention – Taken as an adjunct to diet, exercise, and smoking cessation, statins can reduce the risk of first cardiovascular events and death in patients at increased risk for atherosclerotic cardiovascular disease (ASCVD).[2] Even in patients at moderate risk, treatment with a statin reduces the incidence of cardiovascular events significantly more than placebo.[3]

Choice of a Lipid-Lowering Drug

▸ Statins are the lipid-lowering drugs of choice for treatment of hyperlipidemia and for prevention of cardiovascular disease in most patients.

▸ Statins can reduce the risk of a first cardiovascular event and death in patients at increased risk for atherosclerotic cardiovascular disease (ASCVD).

▸ Statins can decrease the risk of major coronary events and death in patients with ASCVD.

▸ Addition of ezetimibe to a statin can reduce the risk of secondary cardiovascular events.

▸ Addition of a PCSK9 inhibitor to a statin can reduce LDL-C levels much more than a statin alone and can reduce the risk of secondary cardiovascular events.

▸ Limited evidence suggests that use of a bile acid sequestrant alone or in combination with a statin may reduce the risk of cardiovascular events.

▸ Gemfibrozil is the only fibrate with demonstrated beneficial effects on cardiovascular outcomes, but its use with statins can increase the risk of myopathy and is not recommended.

▸ There is no convincing evidence that adding extended-release niacin to a statin improves cardiovascular outcomes.

▸ Icosapent ethyl, an omega-3 polyunsaturated fatty acid, reduced the risk of ischemic cardiovascular events in patients with hypertriglyceridemia and cardiac risk factors in one randomized controlled trial.

Secondary Prevention – Controlled trials in patients with previous cardiovascular events have shown that high-intensity statin therapy decreases the incidence of cardiac events, stroke, and cardiovascular death significantly more than less intensive statin regimens.[4]

In one meta-analysis of 26 trials (including both primary and secondary prevention trials) in about 170,000 patients, each 1 mmol/L (39 mg/dL) reduction in LDL-C was associated with a 22% reduction in major vascular events and a 10% reduction in all-cause mortality.[5]

Adverse Effects – All statins are generally well tolerated.[6] Some patients who cannot tolerate one statin may tolerate another.

In clinical practice, muscle pain and weakness with or without increased creatine kinase (CK) levels are often reported in patients taking statins, but in randomized trials, muscle symptoms may occur equally often in patients taking placebo.[7,8] CK levels should be measured at baseline and again if myalgia occurs. Most cases of CK elevation are mild to moderate in severity and can be managed by reducing the dose or switching to a less potent statin. Rarely, rhabdomyolysis and myoglobinemia leading to renal failure can occur.

An increase in serum aminotransferase levels to >3 times the upper limit of normal (ULN) occurs in 1-2% of patients receiving high-intensity statin therapy, but whether statins actually cause liver damage is unclear.

Statin therapy has been associated with an increased incidence of new-onset diabetes, particularly in patients with diabetes risk factors. In all patients, including those at high risk for diabetes, the cardiovascular and mortality benefits of statin therapy far outweigh the risk of developing diabetes.[9]

Some reports have suggested an association between use of statins and cancer, but in one meta-analysis of 26 trials that included about 170,000 patients followed for ≥2 years, there was no correlation between the use or intensity of statin therapy and the incidence of cancer or nonvascular death.[5]

An increased incidence of hemorrhagic stroke has been associated with statin therapy in some trials, but in one meta-analysis of 31 trials, patients taking a statin had similar hemorrhagic stroke rates and significantly lower total stroke and all-cause mortality rates than those not taking a statin.[10]

Peripheral neuropathy, memory loss, sleep disturbances, erectile dysfunction, gynecomastia, a lupus-like syndrome, and acute pancreatitis have been reported with statin use, but there is no convincing evidence of causal relationships.

Drug Interactions – Statin-induced myopathy can be precipitated by drug interactions.[11] Simvastatin and lovastatin undergo extensive first-pass metabolism by CYP3A4; concurrent use of a strong CYP3A4 inhibitor can increase their serum concentrations dramatically. Atorvastatin undergoes less first-pass metabolism by CYP3A4, but rhabdomyolysis has occurred with concurrent use of CYP3A4 inhibitors. Grapefruit juice inhibits CYP3A; patients taking atorvastatin, lovastatin, or simvastatin should avoid consuming large amounts (>1 L/day) of grapefruit juice. Fluvastatin is metabolized primarily by CYP2C9; concurrent use of a CYP2C9 inhibitor could increase the risk of myopathy. Pravastatin, rosuvastatin, and pitavastatin are not metabolized to a clinically significant extent by CYP isozymes.

Transporter proteins such as organic anion transporter polypeptides (OATP), P-glycoprotein (P-gp), and breast cancer resistance protein (BCRP) may play a role in statin pharmacokinetics; statins should be used with caution with drugs that inhibit these transporters.[12,13]

Concurrent administration of cyclosporine (*Neoral*, and others) increases serum concentrations of all statins and the risk of rhabdomyolysis, probably through inhibition of CYP3A4, OATP, and P-gp. Concurrent use of gemfibrozil (*Lopid*, and generics) can increase statin concentrations and the risk of rhabdomyolysis, possibly through inhibition of OATP, and is not recommended. In patients taking dabigatran etexilate *(Pradaxa),* concurrent use of simvastatin or lovastatin may increase the risk of major hemorrhage; the mechanism for this interaction is unclear.[14]

Bile acid sequestrants can interfere with the absorption of statins; they should be taken several hours before or after statins. Colesevelam does not appear to interfere with the absorption of most statins.

Pregnancy and Lactation – All statins are contraindicated for use during pregnancy and while breastfeeding; fetal anomalies have been reported in infants whose mothers took the drugs during pregnancy.

Choice of a Statin — All FDA-approved statins have been shown to reduce cardiovascular risk; the magnitude of the reduction is related to the magnitude of LDL-C lowering.[15] Atorvastatin and rosuvastatin at their highest approved doses are the most effective in lowering LDL-C levels and their beneficial effects on clinical outcomes are well-documented.

All of the statins except pitavastatin and pitavastatin magnesium are available generically.[16,17] Dosage adjustments are not required with atorvastatin or fluvastatin in patients with severe renal impairment. Pravastatin, rosuvastatin, and pitavastatin are not metabolized by CYP isozymes and are less likely to interact with other drugs.

CHOLESTEROL ABSORPTION INHIBITOR — Ezetimibe (*Zetia*, and generics) inhibits intestinal absorption of dietary and biliary cholesterol by blocking its transport at the brush border of the small intestine. It reduces LDL-C levels by about 20-25%. The fixed-dose combination of ezetimibe and simvastatin (*Vytorin*, and generics) reduces LDL-C levels more than simvastatin alone. In a large, long-term (median follow-up of 6 years) secondary prevention trial (IMPROVE-IT), adding ezetimibe 10 mg/day to simvastatin 40 mg/day resulted in a statistically significant reduction in cardiovascular events compared to adding placebo.[18]

Adverse Effects – Ezetimibe is generally well tolerated. Diarrhea, arthralgia, rhabdomyolysis, hepatitis, pancreatitis, and thrombocytopenia have been reported, but causal relationships are unclear. In the IMPROVE-IT trial, the incidence of adverse events with ezetimibe plus a statin was similar to that with a statin alone.[18] Patients with moderate to severe hepatic impairment should not take ezetimibe.

Drug Interactions – Ezetimibe may increase the anticoagulant effect of warfarin. Concurrent use of ezetimibe and cyclosporine increases serum concentrations of both drugs. Concurrent use of gemfibrozil and ezetimibe can increase the risk of cholelithiasis and is contraindicated. Bile acid sequestrants interfere with the absorption of ezetimibe; they should be taken several hours before or after ezetimibe.

Pregnancy and Lactation – Skeletal anomalies were detected in the offspring of rats and rabbits given 10-150 times the usual human dose of ezetimibe. The drug has been detected in the milk of lactating rats. There are no data on the presence of ezetimibe in human breast milk or on its effects on the breastfed infant or milk production.

Table 1. 2018 ACC/AHA Task Force Recommendations[1]

Primary Prevention

Patients with LDL-C ≥190 mg/dL
High-intensity statin therapy[2] to a goal of LDL-C <100 mg/dL, if necessary adding ezetimibe and then (if multiple ASCVD risk factors are present) possibly a PCSK9 inhibitor

Patients 40-75 years old with diabetes and LDL-C ≥70 mg/dL
Moderate-intensity statin therapy[3]

Patients with diabetes and LDL-C ≥70 mg/dL who have multiple risk factors or age 50-75 years
High-intensity statin therapy[2] to reduce LDL-C ≥50%

Patients 40-75 years old without diabetes, LDL-C ≥70 mg/dL, and 10-year ASCVD risk <20%[4]
Consider LDL-C level and risk-enhancing factors[5] in decision to start moderate-intensity statin therapy[3] to reduce LDL-C 30-49%

Patients 40-75 years old without diabetes, LDL-C ≥70 mg/dL, and 10-year ASCVD risk ≥20%[4]
High-intensity statin therapy[2] to reduce LDL-C ≥50%

Patients >75 years old
Consider risks and benefits

Secondary Prevention

Patients with clinical ASCVD[6]
High-intensity[2] or maximally tolerated statin therapy to reduce LDL-C ≥50%

Patients with very high-risk ASCVD (multiple major ASCVD events[7] or one major ASCVD event and multiple high-risk conditions[8])
Maximally tolerated statin therapy to a goal of LDL-C <70 mg/dL, if necessary adding ezetimibe and then possibly a PCSK9 inhibitor

ASCVD = atherosclerotic cardiovascular disease
1. Adapted from SM Grundy et al. J Am Coll Cardiol 2018 November 10 (epub).
2. **High-intensity** statin therapy (atorvastatin 40-80 mg/day, rosuvastatin 20-40 mg/day) lowers LDL-C ≥50%.
3. **Moderate-intensity** statin therapy (e.g. atorvastatin 10-20 mg/day, rosuvastatin 5-10 mg/day, simvastatin 20-40 mg/day) lowers LDL-C 30-49%.
4. ASCVD Risk Calculator Plus. Available at: http://bit.ly/2ShGUJ0 (DM Lloyd-Jones et al. J Am Coll Cardiol 2018 November 10 epub).
5. **Risk-enhancing factors** include family history of premature ASCVD, persistently elevated LDL-C ≥160 mg/dL, chronic kidney disease, metabolic syndrome, history of preeclampsia or premature menopause, chronic inflammatory diseases, high-risk ethnicity, persistently elevated triglycerides (≥175 mg/dL), and in selected individuals, apolipoprotein B ≥130 mg/dL, high-sensitivity C-reactive protein ≥2.0 mg/L, ankle brachial index <0.9, and lipoprotein(a) ≥50 mg/dL.
6. **Clinical ASCVD** includes acute coronary syndrome, history of myocardial infarction, stable or unstable angina, coronary or other arterial revascularization, stroke, transient ischemic attack, or peripheral artery disease, including aortic aneurysm, all of atherosclerotic origin.
7. **Major ASCVD events** include recent acute coronary syndrome (within the past 12 months), history of myocardial infarction or ischemic stroke, and symptomatic peripheral arterial disease.
8. **High-risk conditions** include age ≥65 years, heterozygous familial hypercholesterolemia, history of prior coronary artery bypass surgery or PCI outside of major ASCVD events, diabetes, hypertension, eGFR 15-59 mL/min/1.73 m², smoking, LDL-C ≥100 mg/dL despite maximally tolerated statin therapy and ezetimibe, and history of heart failure.

PCSK9 INHIBITORS — Alirocumab *(Praluent)* and evolocumab *(Repatha)* are subcutaneously injected monoclonal antibodies that bind to proprotein convertase subtilisin/kexin type 9 (PCSK9) and prevent it from binding to LDL receptors, thereby increasing the number of receptors and clearance of circulating LDL-C.[19,20]

Efficacy – Adding alirocumab or evolocumab to a statin reduces LDL-C levels by 50-60%.[21,22] In a double-blind trial (ODYSSEY OUTCOMES), 18,924 patients who had a recent (1-12 months) acute coronary syndrome and were receiving high-intensity or maximally tolerated statin therapy were randomized to receive **alirocumab** or placebo every 2 weeks. After a median follow-up of 34 months, a composite of death from coronary heart disease, nonfatal myocardial infarction, fatal or nonfatal ischemic stroke, or unstable angina requiring hospitalization, the primary endpoint, occurred in significantly fewer patients treated with alirocumab than with placebo (9.5% vs 11.1%). Reductions in the primary endpoint were greater in patients with baseline LDL-C levels ≥100 mg/dL. Death from any cause occurred in 334 patients (3.5%) with alirocumab and in 392 (4.1%) with placebo.[23]

In a double-blind trial (FOURIER), 27,564 patients with ASCVD and an LDL-C level ≥70 mg/dL who were receiving moderate- or high-intensity statin therapy were randomized to receive **evolocumab** or placebo. Evolocumab reduced the median LDL-C level from 92 to 30 mg/dL. After a median follow-up of 26 months, a composite of cardiovascular death, myocardial infarction, stroke, hospitalization for unstable angina, or coronary revascularization, the primary endpoint, occurred in significantly fewer patients treated with evolocumab than with placebo (9.8% vs 11.3%). There was no significant difference between the two groups in rates of cardiovascular mortality (1.8% with evolocumab vs 1.7% with placebo) or all-cause mortality (3.2% with evolocumab vs 3.1% with placebo).[24]

Adverse Effects – Both alirocumab and evolocumab appear to be well tolerated. Muscle aches, rash, urticaria, and mild injection-site reactions have been reported. No increase in the risk of cognitive adverse events has been observed with either drug compared to placebo in clinical trials.[25,26] Although PCSK9 inhibitors can cause abnormally low LDL-C levels (<25 mg/dL), no associated adverse events have been reported.

Pregnancy and Lactation – A few studies have suggested an association between PCSK9 inhibitor use by women during pregnancy and neural tube defects in their offspring.[27,28] Monoclonal antibodies are unlikely to cross the placenta in the first trimester, but may do so subsequently. Whether alirocumab or evolocumab is present in human breast milk is not known, but human IgG antibodies cross the placenta and can be found in breast milk.

BILE ACID SEQUESTRANTS — The resins cholestyramine (*Questran*, and others) and colestipol (*Colestid*, and generics) and the hydrophilic polymer colesevelam hydrochloride (*Welchol*, and generics) prevent reabsorption of bile acids, resulting in increased conversion of cholesterol to bile acids, depletion of intrahepatic cholesterol, and upregulation of LDL receptor synthesis. These drugs can lower LDL-C levels by up to 20% and increase HDL-C levels, but they may further increase plasma triglyceride levels in patients with hypertriglyceridemia; they should not be used if triglyceride levels are >300 mg/dL. Limited evidence suggests that use of a bile acid sequestrant alone or in combination with a statin may reduce the risk of cardiovascular events.[29]

Adverse Effects – Constipation occurs frequently with colestipol and cholestyramine and may be accompanied by heartburn, nausea, eructation, and bloating. Colesevelam is better tolerated.

Drug Interactions – Bile acid sequestrants can interfere with the absorption of other oral drugs, including statins and ezetimibe; they should be taken several hours before or after other drugs. Colesevelam does not appear to interfere with the absorption of most statins. These drugs can also interfere with the absorption of fat-soluble vitamins.

Pregnancy and Lactation – Bile acid sequestrants may interfere with maternal absorption of vitamins. Colesevelam did not cause maternal or fetal toxicity in animal studies. Cholestyramine, colestipol, and colesevelam are not absorbed systemically and are not expected to be found in human breast milk.

FIBRIC ACID DERIVATIVES — Fibrates activate the nuclear transcription factor peroxisome proliferator-activated receptor-alpha (PPAR-alpha), which regulates genes that control lipid and glucose metabolism, inflammation, and endothelial function. Gemfibrozil (*Lopid*, and generics), fenofibrate (*Fenoglide*, and others), fenofibric acid (*Fibricor*, and others), and bezafibrate (not available in the US) decrease triglyceride and VLDL-C levels, usually by 25-50%, and may increase HDL-C levels. They may decrease LDL-C levels in patients with low to normal triglycerides, but may increase LDL-C levels when they are used to treat elevated triglycerides. Patients with hypertriglyceridemia (persistently above 886 mg/dL) severe enough to increase the risk of pancreatitis should be treated with a fibrate.[30]

Efficacy – Gemfibrozil is the only fibrate with demonstrated beneficial effects on cardiovascular outcomes,[31] but its use with statins can increase the risk of myopathy and is not recommended. Fenofibrate may be more effective than gemfibrozil in lowering LDL-C and triglyceride levels; there is no evidence, however, that addition of fenofibrate to a statin improves cardiovascular outcomes.[32,33]

Fenofibric acid is no longer FDA-approved for use with a statin to reduce triglyceride levels and increase HDL-C levels.[34]

Adverse Effects – Gastrointestinal adverse effects are common with fibrates. Cholelithiasis, hepatitis, and myositis can occur. A paradoxical severe decrease in HDL-C levels has been reported; if this occurs, the fibrate should be stopped. Fibrates are contraindicated in patients with liver or gallbladder disease. Fenofibrate can increase serum creatinine levels; the dose should be reduced in patients with mild to moderate renal impairment and fenofibrate should not be used in those with severe renal impairment.

Table 2. Some Lipid-Lowering Drugs

Drug	Some Formulations
Statins	
Atorvastatin – generic Lipitor (Pfizer)	10, 20, 40, 80 mg tabs
Fluvastatin – generic Lescol (Novartis)	20, 40 mg caps
extended-release – generic Lescol XL	80 mg ER tabs
Lovastatin – generic	10, 20, 40 mg tabs
extended-release – Altoprev (Covis)	20, 40, 60 mg ER tabs
Pitavastatin calcium[6] – Livalo (Kowa)	1, 2, 4 mg tabs
Pitavastatin magnesium[6] – Zypitamag (Medicure)	1, 2, 4 mg tabs
Pravastatin – generic Pravachol (BMS)	10, 20, 40, 80 mg tabs 20, 40, 80 mg tabs
Rosuvastatin – generic Crestor (AstraZeneca)	5, 10, 20, 40 mg tabs

Simvastatin – generic
  Zocor (Merck)
  Flolipid (Salerno)
	5, 10, 20, 40, 80 mg tabs
	10, 20, 40, 80 mg tabs
	20 mg/5 mL, 40 mg/5 mL susp

susp = suspension

1. FDA-approved dosage. Some expert clinicians use lower doses for initial treatment of patients with only modest elevations of LDL-C or a history of poor tolerance to these drugs. For patients who require a large reduction in LDL-C, some would use higher doses initially. Statins are generally most effective when taken in the evening. Dosage adjustments may be needed for patients with renal or hepatic impairment.
2. The listed ranges correspond to the initial and maximum dosages. Statin regimens that lower LDL-C ≥50% are considered high-intensity therapy. Those that lower LDL-C 30-49% are considered moderate-intensity therapy, and those that lower LDL-C <30% are considered low-intensity therapy. LDL-C reductions may vary significantly among individuals.
3. Approximate WAC for 30 days' treatment with the lowest usual initial adult dosage. WAC = wholesaler acquisition cost or manufacturer's published price to wholesalers; WAC represents a published catalogue or list price and may not represent an actual transactional price. Source: AnalySource® Monthly. January 5, 2019. Reprinted with permission by First Databank, Inc. All rights reserved. ©2019. www.fdbhealth.com/policies/drug-pricing-policy.

Usual Adult Dosage[1]	Average LDL-C Reduction[2]	Cost[3]
Initial: 10-20 mg once/day	35-40%	$5.60
Maximum: 80 mg once/day	50-60%	299.40
Initial: 40 mg bid	30-35%	220.10
Maximum: 40 mg bid	30-35%	306.00
Initial: 80 mg once/day	35-40%	194.10
Maximum: 80 mg once/day	35-40%	323.00
Initial: 20 mg once/day	25-30%	6.30
Maximum: 80 mg once/day[4,5]	35-40%	
Initial: 20 mg once/day	20-25%	921.10
Maximum: 60 mg once/day[5]	40-45%	
Initial: 2 mg once/day[7]	35-40%	
Maximum: 4 mg once/day[7]	40-45%	295.60
Initial: 2 mg once/day[7]	35-40%	
Maximum: 4 mg once/day[7]	40-45%	232.50
Initial: 40 mg once/day[8]	30-35%	14.20
Maximum: 80 mg once/day	35-40%	169.70
Initial: 10-20 mg once/day[9,10]	45-50%	11.80
Maximum: 40 mg once/day[10,11]	50-60%	260.90
Initial: 10-20 mg once/day[12]	35-40%	3.20
Maximum: 40 mg once/day[13,14]	45-50%	138.60
		121.70

4. Or 40 mg bid.
5. Use doses >20 mg/day cautiously in patients with severe renal impairment.
6. The FDA considers *Livalo* and *Zypitamag* to be bioequivalent.
7. 1 mg/day initially, 2 mg/day maximum in patients with moderate or severe renal impairment.
8. 10 mg initially for patients with severe renal impairment.
9. Higher serum concentrations of rosuvastatin have been reported in Asian patients; an initial dose of 5 mg once daily is recommended.
10. Patients with severe renal impairment not on hemodialysis should start with 5 mg and not exceed 10 mg/day.
11. Maximum dose is 20 mg/day in Asian patients (E Lee et al. Clin Pharmacol 2005; 78:330).
12. Patients with severe renal impairment should start with 5 mg.
13. Patients who have taken 80 mg/day of simvastatin for ≥12 months without evidence of myopathy can continue at this dose.
14. The maximum dose of simvastatin is 10 mg if taken with diltiazem, dronedarone, or verapamil and 20 mg if taken with amiodarone, amlodipine, or ranolazine.

Continued on next page

Table 2. Some Lipid-Lowering Drugs (continued)

Drug	Some Formulations
Cholesterol Absorption Inhibitor	
Ezetimibe – generic *Zetia* (Merck)	10 mg tabs
Cholesterol Absorption Inhibitor/Statin Combination	
Ezetimibe/simvastatin – generic *Vytorin* (Merck)	10/10, 10/20, 10/40, 10/80 mg tabs
PCSK9 Inhibitors	
Alirocumab – *Praluent* (Sanofi/Regeneron)	75, 150 mg/mL single-use prefilled pens
Evolocumab – *Repatha* (Amgen)	140 mg/mL single-use prefilled syringes
Repatha Sureclick	140 mg/mL single-use prefilled autoinjectors
Repatha Pushtronex	420 mg/3.5 mL single-use infusors with prefilled cartridges
Bile Acid Sequestrants	
Colesevelam – generic *Welchol* (Daiichi Sankyo)	625 mg tabs; 3.75 g packets
Colestipol – generic *Colestid* (Pfizer)	1 g tabs; 5 g packets; 5 g/scoop 1 g tabs; 5, 7.5 g packets; 5 g/scoop
Cholestyramine – generic *Questran* (Par)	4 g packets; 4 g/scoop
Cholestyramine light[24] – generic *Prevalite* (Upsher-Smith)	4 g packets; 4 g/scoop

15. The 300-mg dose is given as 2 consecutive 150-mg injections at different sites.
16. Alone or when added to statin therapy.
17. Cost of one pen, syringe, autoinjector, or infusor with cartridge.
18. Dosage for patients with heterozygous familial hypercholesterolemia (HeFH) or atherosclerotic cardiovascular disease (ASCVD). Dosage for patients with homozygous familial hypercholesterolemia (HoFH) is 420 mg SC once monthly.
19. The 420-mg dose is given as a single dose through the infusor or as three consecutive 140-mg injections within 30 minutes.

Usual Adult Dosage[1]	Average LDL-C Reduction[2]	Cost[3]
10 mg once/day	20-25%	$36.80
		345.00
Initial: 10/10-10/20 mg once/day	40-50%	158.90
Maximum: 10/40 mg once/day[13,14]	50-60%	341.70
Initial: 75 mg SC q2 wks	45-50%[16]	560.00[17]
or 300 mg SC q4 wks[15]	50-60%[16]	
Maximum: 150 mg SC q2 wks		
or 300 mg SC q4 wks[15]		
Initial: 140 mg SC q2 wks or	55-60%[16]	225.00[17]
420 mg SC once/month[18,19]		
Maximum: 420 mg SC once/month[19]		225.00[17]
		487.50[17]
3.75 g once/day or 1.875 g bid[20]	15-20%	561.50[21]
		657.00[21]
10 g once/d or 5 g bid[22]	15-20%	188.70[21]
or 2-16 g once/d or divided[23]		442.10[21]
8 g once/d or 4 g bid	15-20%	122.30[21]
		341.20[21]
		123.00[21]
		123.00[21]

20. Should be taken with food.
21. Cost of a 30-day supply of packets.
22. Dosage for granules.
23. Dosage for tablets.
24. Contains aspartame instead of sucrose.

Continued on next page

Table 2. Some Lipid-Lowering Drugs (continued)

Drug	Some Formulations
Fibric Acid Derivatives	
Gemfibrozil – generic	600 mg tabs
Lopid (Pfizer)	
Fenofibrate – nonmicronized	
generic	54, 160 mg tabs
Fenoglide (Santarus)	40, 120 mg tabs
Lipofen (Kowa)	50, 150 mg caps
micronized[26] – generic	43, 67, 134, 200 mg caps
Antara (Lupin)	30, 90 mg caps
nanocrystallized[26] – generic	48, 145 mg tabs
Tricor (AbbVie)	48, 145 mg tabs
Triglide (Casper)	160 mg tabs
Fenofibric acid – generic	35, 105 mg tabs
Fibricor (Aralez)	
delayed-release – generic	45, 135 mg delayed-release caps
Trilipix (AbbVie)	
Niacin	
Niacin immediate-release – generic[27]	500 mg caps; 500 mg tabs
Niacor (Avondale)	500 mg tabs
extended-release – generic	500, 750, 1000 mg ER tabs
Niaspan (AbbVie)	
sustained-release –	
Slo-Niacin (Main Pointe)[27]	250, 500, 750 mg SR tabs
Fish Oil	
Icosapent ethyl – *Vascepa* (Amarin)	500 mg, 1 g caps[29]
Omega-3 acid ethyl esters – generic	1 g caps[31]
Lovaza (GSK)	
Omega-3 carboxylic acids –	
Epanova (Astra Zeneca)	1 g caps[32]

N.A. = Cost not yet available. Product has not yet been marketed.
25. LDL-C levels may increase when triglyceride levels are decreased.
26. Nanocrystallized and micronized formulations may result in greater solubility and improved bioavailability compared to nonmicronized formulations.
27. Available over the counter.
28. Should be taken with a low-fat snack at bedtime.

Usual Adult Dosage[1]	Average LDL-C Reduction[2]	Cost[3]
600 mg bid	5-10%[25]	$6.80
		403.40
	5-10%[25]	
160 mg once/day[20]		62.60
120 mg once/day[20]		1113.20
150 mg once/day[20]		222.90
200 mg once/day[20]		66.20
90 mg once/day		507.90
145 mg once/day		45.80
145 mg once/day		31.00
160 mg once/day		341.90
105 mg once/day	5-10%[25]	72.10
		158.40
135 mg once/day		133.40
		270.70
1000 mg tid	5-25%	4.10
1000-2000 mg bid or tid		388.80
1000-2000 mg once/day[28]		180.00
		274.20
750 mg once/day		14.50
2 g bid[20,30]	0-5%	303.70
4 g once/day or 2 g bid[30]	See footnote 25	129.10
		299.40
2-4 g once/day[30]	See footnote 25	N.A.

29. EPA content.
30. FDA-approved dosage for treating hypertriglyceridemia (≥500 mg/dL).
31. Each 1000-mg capsule contains about 465 mg EPA and about 375 mg DHA (total 900 mg polyunsaturated fatty acids [PUFAs]).
32. Each 1000-mg capsule contains at least 850 mg of PUFAs.

Continued on next page

Table 2. Some Lipid-Lowering Drugs (continued)	
Drug	**Some Formulations**
Fish Oil (continued)	
USP-verified fish oil capsules[33]	1, 1.2 g caps[34]

33. Available over the counter. USP-verified fish oil products are considered dietary supplements and are manufactured by Nature's Bounty, Kirkland Signature, and Nature Made.
34. Most 1-gram capsules contain 300 mg PUFAs (180 mg EPA and 120 mg DHA). Nature Made 1.2-g capsules contain 360 mg PUFAs (216 mg EPA and 144 mg DHA); three capsules are approximately equal to one *Lovaza* capsule.

Drug Interactions – Fibrates may potentiate the effects of warfarin and antihyperglycemic drugs. Gemfibrozil can increase serum concentrations of statins, possibly through inhibition of OATP, increasing the risk of rhabdomyolysis; concurrent use is not recommended. Concurrent use of gemfibrozil and ezetimibe can increase the risk of cholelithiasis and is contraindicated. Fenofibrate is eliminated renally and should be used with caution in patients taking cyclosporine or other nephrotoxic drugs.

Pregnancy and Lactation – Adverse effects on fetal development have been observed with gemfibrozil and fenofibrate in animal studies. There are no data on the presence of fibric acid derivatives in human breast milk or on their effects on the breastfed infant or milk production.

NIACIN — Niacin (nicotinic acid) has favorable effects on all plasma lipoproteins and lipids. Monotherapy increases HDL-C levels by 15-35%, decreases triglyceride levels by 10-50%, and decreases LDL-C levels by 5-25%. It also decreases plasma levels of lipoprotein(a), a marker of cardiovascular risk.[35]

Efficacy – In a meta-analysis of 11 randomized, controlled trials that included 6616 patients, use of niacin was found to have a beneficial effect for secondary prevention of cardiovascular events, but the included trials varied in size and quality.[36] In a trial in patients with ASCVD (HPS2-THRIVE), addition of niacin and the prostaglandin inhibitor laropiprant

Usual Adult Dosage[1]	Average LDL-C Reduction[2]	Cost[3]
4-4.8 g tid	See footnote 25	$19.30[35]

35. Cost of 2 bottles containing 400 Nature Made capsules at costco.com. Accessed January 30, 2019.

(to reduce flushing; no longer available in the US) to statin therapy did not significantly reduce the incidence of first major vascular events and was associated with an increased incidence of diabetes, serious gastrointestinal events, infection, and bleeding.[37] There is no convincing evidence that adding extended-release niacin to a statin improves cardiovascular outcomes; extended-release niacin is no longer FDA-approved for use with a statin for treatment of high cholesterol.[38]

Adverse Effects – Niacin can cause flushing, pruritus, gastrointestinal distress, blurred vision, fatigue, glucose intolerance, hyperuricemia, hepatic toxicity, exacerbation of peptic ulcers and, rarely, dry eyes or skin hyperpigmentation. Some adverse effects, particularly flushing, are more common with the immediate-release formulation. Cutaneous reactions to niacin can be diminished by starting with a low dose that is taken after meals and at least 30 minutes after aspirin (81-325 mg).

Pregnancy and Lactation – Niacin can cross the placenta and is not recommended for use during pregnancy. It is found in human breast milk.

FISH OIL — Long-chain omega-3 polyunsaturated fatty acids (PUFAs) are found in algae and cold-water fish such as herring and salmon. They can reduce elevated fasting triglyceride concentrations by 20-50% by decreasing hepatic triglyceride production and increasing triglyceride clearance.[39] Long-term use may increase HDL-C levels.

Efficacy – Most clinical trials of fish oil supplements do not provide any convincing evidence that they prevent cardiovascular disease or improve outcomes in patients who already have it.[40-42]

A combination of eicosapentaenoic acid and docosa-hexaenoic acid (EPA/DHA; *Lovaza*, and generics), available by prescription, was the first omega-3 PUFA product to be approved by the FDA for treatment of severe hypertriglyceridemia. Daily doses of 3-12 g can lower triglycerides by 20-50%, but have not been shown to prevent pancreatitis, which is a major concern in patients with very high triglycerides. Icosapent ethyl *(Vascepa),* the second prescription omega-3 PUFA product to be approved for treatment of severe hypertriglyceridemia, is the ethyl ester of EPA. In one randomized double-blind trial in patients with hypertriglyceridemia and cardiac risk factors, it reduced triglyceride levels and significantly decreased the incidence of cardiovascular events compared to placebo (17.2% vs 22.0%).[43] *Epanova,* a third omega-3 PUFA prescription product that contains EPA and DHA in free fatty acid form, was approved by the FDA for treatment of severe hypertriglyceridemia, but has not yet been marketed.[44]

Adverse Effects – Fish oil supplements are generally well tolerated. Adverse effects have included eructation, dyspepsia, and an unpleasant aftertaste. Worsening glycemic control has been reported in diabetic patients taking high doses. Inhibition of platelet aggregation and increased bleeding time can occur with high doses of fish oil; whether it can cause clinically significant bleeding has not been established. DHA can increase LDL-C levels, but EPA apparently does not.

Pregnancy and Lactation – Omega-3 PUFAs given at 7 times the recommended human dose were embryocidal in rats. Omega-3 PUFAs are secreted in human breast milk.

HOMOZYGOUS FAMILIAL HYPERCHOLESTEROLEMIA — A rare inherited condition (estimated prevalence 1:300,000 to 1:1,000,000 persons) that is most commonly caused by defects in the LDL receptor gene, homozygous familial hypercholesterolemia (HoFH) causes very high LDL-C levels, cutaneous xanthoma soon after birth, and, without treatment, premature cardiovascular disease and death.

Two drugs are FDA-approved solely for treatment of HoFH: mipomersen *(Kynamro)*, which must be injected subcutaneously and is approved for use in persons ≥12 years old, and lomitapide *(Juxtapid)*, which is taken orally and is approved for use in adults.[45] Both drugs can lower LDL-C (by 25% with mipomersen and 40% with lomitapide) in patients with HoFH already taking maximum dosages of other lipid-lowering drugs.[46] Serious adverse effects, particularly hepatotoxicity, can occur with both drugs. The PCSK9 inhibitor evolocumab *(Repatha)* was also recently approved for treatment of HoFH based on the results of a large randomized trial that showed it reduced LDL-C levels by 31% compared to placebo.[47]

1. SM Grundy et al. 2018 AHA/ACC/AACVPR/AAPA/ABC/ACPM/ADA/AGS/APhA/ ASPC/NLA/PCNA Guideline on the management of blood cholesterol: a report of the American College of Cardiology/American Heart Association task force on clinical practice guidelines. J Am Coll Cardiol 2018 November 3 (epub).
2. R Chou et al. Statins for prevention of cardiovascular disease in adults: evidence report and systematic review for the US Preventive Services Task Force. JAMA 2016; 316:2008.
3. S Yusuf et al. Cholesterol lowering in intermediate-risk persons without cardiovascular disease. N Engl J Med 2016; 374:2021.
4. F Rodriguez et al. Association between intensity of statin therapy and mortality in patients with atherosclerotic cardiovascular disease. JAMA Cardiol 2017; 2:47.
5. CTT Collaboration et al. Efficacy and safety of more intensive lowering of LDL cholesterol: a meta-analysis of data from 170,000 participants in 26 randomised trials. Lancet 2010; 376:1670.
6. CB Newman et al. Statin safety and associated adverse events: a scientific statement from the American Heart Association. Arterioscler Thromb Vasc Biol 2019; 39:e38.
7. A Gupta et al. Adverse events associated with unblinded, but not with blinded, statin therapy in the Anglo-Scandinavian Cardiac Outcomes Trial-Lipid-Lowering Arm (ASCOT-LLA): a randomised double-blind placebo-controlled trial and its non-randomised non-blind extension phase. Lancet 2017; 389:2473.
8. HV Ganga et al. A systematic review of statin-induced muscle problems in clinical trials. Am Heart J 2014; 168:6.
9. PM Ridker et al. Cardiovascular benefits and diabetes risks of statin therapy in primary prevention: an analysis from the JUPITER trial. Lancet 2012; 380:565.
10. JS McKinney and WJ Kostis. Statin therapy and the risk of intracerebral hemorrhage: a meta-analysis of 31 randomized controlled trials. Stroke 2012; 43:2149.

11. Inhibitors and inducers of CYP enzymes and P-glycoprotein. Med Lett Drugs Ther 2017 September 18 (epub). Available at: medicalletter.org/downloads/CYP_PGP_Tables.pdf.

12. R Elsby et al. Solitary inhibition of the breast cancer resistance protein efflux transporter results in a clinically significant drug-drug interaction with rosuvastatin by causing up to a 2-fold increase in statin exposure. Drug Metab Dispos 2016; 44:398.

13. BS Wiggins et al. Recommendations for management of clinically significant drug-drug interactions with statins and select agents used in patients with cardiovascular disease: a scientific statement from the American Heart Association. Circulation 2016; 134:e468.

14. Drug interaction: dabigatran (Pradaxa) and statins. Med Lett Drugs Ther 2017; 59:26.

15. MG Silverman et al. Association between lowering LDL-C and cardiovascular risk reduction among different therapeutic interventions: a systematic review and meta-analysis. JAMA 2016; 316:1289.

16. Pitavastatin (Livalo) – the seventh statin. Med Lett Drugs Ther 2010; 52:64.

17. In brief: Pitavastatin magnesium (Zypitamag) for hyperlipidemia. Med Lett Drugs Ther 2018; 60:106.

18. CP Cannon et al. Ezetimibe added to statin therapy after acute coronary syndromes. N Engl J Med 2015; 372:2387.

19. Alirocumab (Praluent) to lower LDL-cholesterol. Med Lett Drugs Ther 2015; 57:113.

20. Evolocumab (Repatha) – a second PCSK9 inhibitor to lower LDL-cholesterol. Med Lett Drugs Ther 2015; 57:140.

21. JG Robinson et al. Efficacy and safety of alirocumab in reducing lipids and cardiovascular events. N Engl J Med 2015; 372:1489.

22. MS Sabatine et al. Efficacy and safety of evolocumab in reducing lipids and cardiovascular events. N Engl J Med 2015; 372:1500.

23. GG Schwartz et al. Alirocumab and cardiovascular outcomes after acute coronary syndrome. N Engl J Med 2018; 379:2097.

24. MS Sabatine et al. Evolocumab and clinical outcomes in patients with cardiovascular disease. N Engl J Med 2017; 376:1713.

25. RP Giugliano et al. Cognitive function in a randomized trial of evolocumab. N Engl J Med 2017; 377:633.

26. PD Harvey et al. No evidence of neurocognitive adverse events associated with alirocumab treatment in 3340 patients from 14 randomized phase 2 and 3 controlled trials: a meta-analysis of individual patient data. Eur Heart J 2018; 39:374.

27. Z Yuan. Dysregulated expressions of PCSK9 are associated with neural tube defects. Atherosclerosis 2018; 32:143.

28. RN Jerome et al. Using human 'experiments of nature' to predict drug safety issues: an example with PCSK9 inhibitors. Drug Saf 2018; 41:303.

29. S Ross et al. Effect of bile acid sequestrants on the risk of cardiovascular events: a Mendelian randomization analysis. Circ Cardiovasc Genet 2015; 8:618.

30. Drugs for hypertriglyceridemia. Med Lett Drugs Ther 2013; 55:17.

31. HB Rubins et al. Gemfibrozil for the secondary prevention of coronary heart disease in men with low levels of high-density lipoprotein cholesterol. Veterans Affairs High-Density Lipoprotein Cholesterol Intervention Trial Study Group. N Engl J Med 1999; 341:410.

32. The ACCORD Study Group et al. Effects of combination lipid therapy in type 2 diabetes mellitus. N Engl J Med 2010; 362:1563.
33. AB Goldfine et al. Fibrates in the treatment of dyslipidemias – time for a reassessment. N Engl J Med 2011; 365:481.
34. FDA. AbbVie Inc. et al; withdrawal of approval of indications related to the coadministration with statins in applications for niacin extended-release tablets and fenofibric acid delayed-release capsules. Federal Register 2016 April 18; 81 FR 22612. Docket No. FDA-2016-N-1127.
35. P Willeit et al. Baseline and on-statin treatment lipoprotein(a) levels for prediction of cardiovascular events: individual patient-data meta-analysis of statin outcome trials. Lancet 2018; 392:1311.
36. E Bruckert et al. Meta-analysis of the effect of nicotinic acid alone or in combination on cardiovascular events and atherosclerosis. Atherosclerosis 2010; 210:353.
37. HPS2-THRIVE Collaborative Group et al. Effects of extended-release niacin with laropiprant in high-risk patients. N Engl J Med 2014; 371:203.
38. DM Lloyd-Jones. Niacin and HDL cholesterol – time to face facts. N Engl J Med 2014; 371:271.
39. Fish oil supplements. Med Lett Drugs Ther 2012; 54:83.
40. Risk and Prevention Study Collaborative Group et al. N-3 fatty acids in patients with multiple cardiovascular risk factors. N Engl J Med 2013; 368:1800.
41. SM Kwak et al. Efficacy of omega-3 fatty acid supplements (eicosapentaenoic acid and docosahexaenoic acid) in the secondary prevention of cardiovascular disease: a meta-analysis of randomized, double-blind, placebo-controlled trials. Arch Intern Med 2012; 172:686.
42. JE Manson et al. Marine n-3 fatty acids and prevention of cardiovascular disease and cancer. N Engl J Med 2019; 380:23.
43. DL Bhatt et al. Cardiovascular risk reduction with icosapent ethyl for hypertriglyceridemia. N Engl J Med 2019; 380:11.
44. JJ Kastelein et al. Omega-3 free fatty acids for the treatment of severe hypertriglyceridemia: the EpanoVa fOr Lowering Very high triglyceridEs (EVOLVE) trial. J Clin Lipidol 2014; 8:94.
45. DJ Rader and JJ Kastelein. Lomitapide and mipomersen: two first-in-class drugs for reducing low-density lipoprotein cholesterol in patients with homozygous familial hypercholesterolemia. Circulation 2014; 129:1022.
46. Two new drugs for homozygous familial hypercholesterolemia. Med Lett Drugs Ther 2013; 55:25.
47. FJ Raal et al. Inhibition of PCSK9 with evolocumab in homozygous familial hypercholesterolaemia (TESLA Part B): a randomised, double-blind, placebo-controlled trial. Lancet 2015; 385:341.

DRUGS FOR
Psoriasis

Original publication date – June 2019

Mild to moderate psoriasis can be treated with topical drugs or with phototherapy. Patients with moderate to severe disease generally require systemic therapy.

TOPICAL THERAPY

Ointments are generally the most effective topical formulation for treatment of psoriasis. Foams and sprays can be applied to large areas, but the alcohol base used in many of them can cause burning in patients with sensitive skin.

CORTICOSTEROIDS — Topical corticosteroids are widely used for treatment of psoriasis, both alone and in combination with phototherapy or systemic therapy.

Adverse Effects – Local cutaneous adverse effects such as atrophy of the dermis and epidermis, telangiectasias, and irreversible striae can occur when these agents are used for prolonged periods of time or under occlusion, when too much is applied, or when corticosteroid-sensitive areas such as the face and intertriginous regions are treated, but usually not when they are applied to active psoriatic lesions. Superpotent topical corticosteroids, such as clobetasol propionate 0.05%, can cause adrenal

Summary

► Topical corticosteroids are generally used for treatment of mild to moderate disease.
► Topical vitamin D analogs or topical tazarotene can be used as alternatives or in addition to topical corticosteroids.
► UV phototherapy can be used for mild to moderate disease that is widespread or has not responded to topical agents.
► Systemic therapy is recommended for patients with moderate to severe disease.
► Methotrexate is effective for treatment of moderate to severe disease.
► Cyclosporine appears to be at least as effective as methotrexate, but use for more than one year is not recommended.
► Acitretin is effective, but it can cause significant mucocutaneous toxicity.
► Apremilast is an expensive oral alternative.
► Biologic agents appear to be the most effective treatment for moderate to severe disease, but they may lose efficacy over time and they are expensive.
► IL-17A antagonists and IL-23 antagonists have been more effective than some TNF inhibitors or the IL-12/23 antagonist ustekinumab.

suppression when applied to large areas, but clinically significant adrenal insufficiency is rare.

Pregnancy and Lactation – Mild-to-moderate potency topical corticosteroids appear to be safe for use during pregnancy and in women who are breastfeeding.[1]

CALCIPOTRIENE — The synthetic vitamin D analog calcipotriene (*Dovonex*, and others) is about as effective as a medium-potency corticosteroid for topical treatment of plaque psoriasis. UVA exposure can inactivate calcipotriene.[2]

Adverse Effects – Calcipotriene is generally well tolerated, but burning and itching can occur. Hypercalcemia has been reported rarely.

Pregnancy and Lactation – There are no adequate studies on the use of calcipotriene in pregnant women. Skeletal abnormalities have occurred in the offspring of animals given oral calcipotriene. There are no data on the presence of calcipotriene in human breast milk after topical application or its effects on the breastfed infant or milk production.

Calcipotriene/Betamethasone Dipropionate – This combination (*Taclonex,* and others) is more effective than either component alone for treating plaque psoriasis and has been well tolerated.[3]

CALCITRIOL — Calcitriol *(Vectical)*, another vitamin D analog, may also be effective for topical treatment of mild to moderate plaque psoriasis in adults.[4]

Adverse Effects – Calcitriol causes less skin irritation than calcipotriene. Skin discomfort, pruritus, and erythema can occur, but are generally mild.

Pregnancy and Lactation – As with calcipotriene, there are no adequate studies on the use of calcitriol in pregnant women. Skeletal abnormalities have been reported in animal studies. There are no data on the presence of calcitriol in human breast milk after topical administration.

TAZAROTENE — The acetylenic retinoid tazarotene (*Tazorac*, and generics) is effective for topical treatment of psoriasis. The therapeutic effect may persist after treatment is stopped; in one 8-week trial, the effect was sustained for at least 4 weeks after treatment was stopped.[5]

Adverse Effects – Erythema, burning, pruritus, peeling, and an increased risk of sunburn can occur with tazarotene. The cream formulation is better tolerated than the gel, but peeling may be more frequent.

Pregnancy and Lactation – Although systemic absorption of tazarotene is minimal after topical application, the drug is tetratogenic and its use is contraindicated during pregnancy. Confirmation that the patient is not pregnant should be obtained before starting treatment. No data are available on the presence of tazarotene in human breast milk or its effects on the breastfed infant or milk production.

Table 1. Some Topical Nonsteroidal Drugs for Psoriasis[1]

Drug	Some Formulations	Cost[2]
Calcipotriene 0.005%[3] – generic	60, 120 g ointment, cream; 60 mL soln	$297.60
Dovonex (Leo)	60, 120 g cream	732.10
Sorilux (Mayne)	60, 100 g foam	770.70
Calcipotriene/betamethasone dipropionate 0.005%/0.064%[4,5] –		
generic	60, 100 g ointment	644.30
Taclonex (Leo)	60, 100 g ointment; 60, 120 g susp	1037.00
Enstilar (Leo)	60 g foam	1050.30
Calcitriol 3 mcg/g[6] –		
Vectical (Galderma)	100 g ointment	908.60
Tazarotene 0.05% and 0.1%[7] –		
generic[8]	30, 60, 100 g cream	252.80
Tazorac (Allergan)	30, 60 g cream; 30, 100 g gel	398.50
Tazarotene/halobetasol propionate 0.045%/0.01%[9] –		
Duobrii (Bausch)	100 g lotion	825.00

1. For information about topical corticosteroids, see Comparison Table: Some Topical Corticosteroids. Available at: secure.medicalletter.org/downloads/1520d_table.pdf.
2. Approximate WAC for one tube or bottle of the lowest available strength and size. WAC = wholesaler acquisition cost or manufacturer's published price to wholesalers; WAC represents a published catalogue or list price and may not represent an actual transactional price. Source: AnalySource® Monthly. June 5, 2019. Reprinted with permission by First Databank, Inc. All rights reserved. ©2019. www.fdbhealth.com/policies/drug-pricing-policy.
3. Applied twice daily.
4. Applied once daily. Adults should not use more than 100 g of ointment or suspension per week or more than 60 g of foam every 4 days.
5. The ointment and foam can be applied for up to 4 weeks and the topical suspension can be applied for up to 8 weeks.
6. Applied twice daily. Maximum dose 200 g/week.
7. Applied once daily in the evening.
8. Generic is only available in 0.1% strength.
9. Applied once daily. Total dosage should not exceed 50 g/week.

Tazarotene/Corticosteroids – Use of tazarotene in combination with a topical corticosteroid may improve its efficacy and tolerability.[6]

CALCINEURIN INHIBITORS — Topical **tacrolimus** (*Protopic,* and generics) and **pimecrolimus** (*Elidel,* and generics) are not FDA-approved for treatment of psoriasis, but they have been shown to be effective for treatment of psoriasis involving the face and intertriginous areas.[7] They can be used as alternatives to topical corticosteroids in such patients.

Adverse Effects – The most common adverse effects of topical calcineurin inhibitors are erythema, burning, and pruritus; they occur less frequently with pimecrolimus. Lymphoma and cutaneous malignancies have been reported rarely in patients who have used topical calcineurin inhibitors; a boxed warning in their labels states that continuous long-term use is not recommended.

Pregnancy and Lactation – There are no adequate studies on the use of topical tacrolimus or pimecrolimus in pregnant women or in women who are breastfeeding. The potential for maternal systemic absorption of these drugs following topical administration is low.[1,8]

PHOTOTHERAPY

UV phototherapy can be used for widespread disease or when psoriasis is unresponsive to topical agents. Narrow-band UVB is safer and more effective than broad-band UVB and has largely replaced it. Oral or topical psoralens combined with UVA radiation (PUVA) is also effective for treating psoriasis, but it can increase the risk of skin cancer. Studies comparing narrow-band UVB with oral or topical PUVA have not shown that either one is consistently more effective than the other for treatment of psoriasis.[9] Excimer laser therapy has been safe and effective for localized disease and is FDA-approved for this indication.[10]

Adverse Effects – Itching, burning, blistering, stinging, dryness, and erythema can occur.

Pregnancy and Lactation – Narrow-band UVB and the excimer laser are considered safe for use during pregnancy.[1] Breastfeeding should be avoided for at least 24 hours after PUVA; UVB phototherapy is preferred for women who are breastfeeding.[8]

SYSTEMIC THERAPY

A variety of drugs, including immunosuppressive agents, retinoids, and biologics, are used for systemic treatment of psoriasis. Their effectiveness is usually measured in clinical trials by a PASI 75 or 90 response (≥75% or ≥90% improvement in Psoriasis Area and Severity Index score). Biologic agents appear to be the most effective, but they are also the most expensive and direct comparisons are limited.[11]

METHOTREXATE — For control of moderate to severe psoriasis refractory to topical therapy, low doses of methotrexate (7.5-25 mg/week), given orally or by SC or IM injection, are often used. In a randomized, double-blind trial of SC methotrexate (17.5-22.5 mg/week) in 120 patients, a PASI 75 reponse was achieved at week 16 in 41% of patients who received methotrexate, compared to 10% of those who received placebo.[12]

Adverse Effects – In low doses, methotrexate is usually well tolerated, but it can cause stomatitis, anorexia, nausea, vomiting, abdominal cramps, fatigue, aminotransferase elevations, and hepatic fibrosis. The GI adverse effects associated with oral methotrexate formulations are less likely to occur with parenteral administration. Hepatotoxicity is the most frequent serious adverse effect; the drug is contraindicated in patients with alcoholism. Methotrexate-induced pneumonitis is rare, but can be fatal. Macrocytic anemia, leukopenia, and thrombocytopenia can occur. Decreased renal function and inadvertent overdosing (daily rather than weekly) are common causes of hematologic toxicity.

Methotrexate is immunosuppressive and should not be used in patients with active infections. In an observational cohort study including 107,707 patients who were new users of systemic drugs for psoriasis, the rate of overall serious infection was higher with methotrexate than with apremilast, etanercept, or ustekinumab, but not different from the rates with acitretin, adalimumab, or infliximab, except for a significant increase in the risk of cellulitis with acitretin.[13]

Drug Interactions – Trimethoprim and other drugs that interfere with folate metabolism may increase bone marrow suppression caused by methotrexate. Proton pump inhibitors (PPIs) and drugs that reduce renal function, particularly NSAIDs, may increase serum concentrations of methotrexate and possibly its toxicity. Concurrent use of methotrexate with alcohol or hepatotoxic drugs, such as acitretin, may increase the risk of hepatotoxicity.

Pregnancy and Lactation – Methotrexate is teratogenic and abortifacient; it is contraindicated for use during pregnancy. After stopping the drug, men should wait a minimum of 3 months and women should probably wait 6 months before attempting to conceive. Methotrexate has been detected in human breast milk; it is contraindicated for use in women who are breastfeeding.

CYCLOSPORINE — Low doses (3-5 mg/kg/day) of cyclosporine (*Neoral*, and others) have been at least as effective as methotrexate for treatment of moderate to severe psoriasis.[14,15]

Adverse Effects – The doses of cyclosporine used for psoriasis have generally been safe, but nephrotoxicity and hypertension can occur; use of the drug for more than one year is not recommended. Cyclosporine can also cause GI disturbances, infection, hirsutism, pruritus, headache, paresthesias, hypertriglyceridemia, and musculoskeletal or joint pain. It can increase the risk of skin malignancies in patients previously treated with PUVA.

Drug Interactions – Use of cyclosporine with other nephrotoxic drugs, such as aminoglycosides, can result in additive nephrotoxic effects. Concurrent use of potassium-sparing diuretics such as spironolactone (*Aldactone*, and generics) with cyclosporine may increase the risk of hyperkalemia. Cyclosporine is a substrate and an inhibitor of CYP3A4 and P-glycoprotein (P-gp); use with CYP3A4 and/or P-gp inhibitors may increase its toxicity and use with inducers may decrease its effectiveness.[16]

Drugs for Psoriasis

Table 2. Some Systemic Drugs for Psoriasis

Drug

Retinoid

Acitretin – generic
 Soriatane (Stiefel)

Phosphodiesterase 4 (PDE4) Inhibitor

Apremilast – *Otezla* (Celgene)

Immunosuppressants

Cyclosporine – generic
 Neoral (Novartis)
 Gengraf (Abbvie)

Methotrexate, oral – generic

Methotrexate, injectable – generic
 Otrexup[5] (Antares)
 Rasuvo[5] (Medac)

TNF Inhibitors

Adalimumab – *Humira*[6,7] (Abbvie)

Certolizumab pegol – *Cimzia* (UCB)

Etanercept – *Enbrel*[10] (Amgen)

Infliximab – *Remicade* (Janssen)
 Infliximab-abda – *Renflexis*[13] (Merck)
 Infliximab-dyyb – *Inflectra*[13] (Pfizer)

IL-12/23 Antagonist

Ustekinumab – *Stelara* (Janssen)

1. Dosage adjustment may be needed for renal or hepatic impairment.
2. Approximate WAC for 3 months' treatment at the lowest usual adult maintenance dosage (cost of starting doses are not included). Cyclosporine and infliximab costs calculated for a patient weighing 80 kg. WAC = wholesaler acquisition cost or manufacturer's published price to wholesalers; WAC represents a published catalogue or list price and may not represent an actual transactional price. Source: AnalySource® Monthly. June 5, 2019. Reprinted with permission by First Databank, Inc. All rights reserved. ©2019. www.fdbhealth.com/policies/drug-pricing-policy.
3. Some expert clinicians recommend not exceeding 25 mg/day to avoid adverse effects.
4. The recommended starting dose is 10 mg, which should be titrated over 5 days to 30 mg to reduce the risk of GI adverse effects. Following the titration, the maintenance dosage is 30 mg bid, which should be reduced to 30 mg once/day in patients with severe renal impairment (CrCl <30 mL/min).
5. Available as single-dose auto-injectors.
6. Four biosimilars, adalimumab-atto *(Amjevita)*, adalimumab-adbm *(Cyltezo)*, adalimumab-adaz *(Hyrimoz)*, and adalimumab-bwwd *(Hadlima)* are FDA-approved, but not yet available.

Usual Adult Dosage[1]	Cost[2]
10-50 mg PO once/day[3]	$1778.40
	3954.10
30 mg PO bid[4]	10,194.00
2.5-5 mg/kg/day PO in 2 divided doses	1416.20
	1536.00
	1253.30
7.5-25 mg/week PO in a single dose or in 3 divided doses over 36 hours	86.30
10-25 mg SC or IM once/week	17.50
10-25 mg SC once/week	1949.40
10-25 mg SC once/week	1479.00
80 mg SC at week 0, 40 mg at week 1, then 40 mg q2 weeks[8]	15,522.30
400 mg SC q2 weeks[9]	25,964.60
50 mg SC twice/week x 12 weeks, then once/week	15,522.20
5 mg/kg IV at weeks 0, 2, and 6, then q8 weeks[11]	9342.60[12]
	5843.10[12]
	7570.20[12]
45 mg or 90 mg[14] SC at weeks 0 and 4, then q12 weeks	11,002.30

7. *Humira Citrate-free* does not contain citrate buffers, which have been associated with injection-site pain (P Nash et al. Rheumatol Ther 2016; 3:257). Other differences compared to original *Humira* include a smaller needle and smaller injection volume.
8. Some patients may require a dose of 40 mg per week for adequate disease control.
9. An alternative regimen for patients weighing ≤90 kg is 400 mg SC at weeks 0, 2, and 4, then 200 mg q2 weeks.
10. Two biosimilars, etanercept-szzs *(Erelzi) and* etanercept-ykro *(Eticovo)*, have been approved by the FDA, but are not yet available.
11. Some patients may require more frequent dosing (every 4 or 6 weeks) and/or a higher dose (10 mg/kg) for adequate disease control.
12. Cost based on two 400-mg doses for infliximab and two 100-mg doses for guselkumab.
13. Biosimilar of infliximab.
14. Dose is 45 mg for patients weighing ≤100 kg and 90 mg for those weighing >100 kg.

Continued on next page

Table 2. Some Systemic Drugs for Psoriasis (continued)
Drug
IL-17A Antagonists[15]
Brodalumab[16] – *Siliq* (Bausch Health)
Ixekizumab – *Taltz* (Lilly)
Secukinumab – *Cosentyx* (Novartis)
IL-23 Antagonists
Guselkumab – *Tremfya* (Janssen)
Risankizumab-rzaa – *Skyrizi* (Abbvie)
Tildrakizumab-asmn – *Ilumya* (Sun)

15. Brodalumab targets the IL-17A receptor. Ixekizumab and secukinumab target IL-17A.
16. Brodalumab is only available through a REMS program because suicidal ideation and behavior, including completed suicides, have occurred in patients treated with the drug.
17. For some patients, 150 mg may be sufficient.

Pregnancy and Lactation – Cyclosporine appears to be relatively safe for use during pregnancy, but it has been associated with low birth weight and prematurity.[1] Cyclosporine is present in human breast milk and detectable levels have been reported in breastfed infants whose mothers were taking the drug.

ACITRETIN — Use of the oral retinoid acitretin (*Soriatane*, and generics) in doses of 25-50 mg/day can reduce the area and severity of psoriasis, but it can cause significant mucocutaneous toxicity. Some expert clinicians recommend using lower doses to avoid adverse effects. Acitretin is often used in combination with UVB radiation or with PUVA.[9]

Adverse Effects – Like other oral retinoids, acitretin can cause dose-related cheilitis, hair loss, dry skin, and desquamation. Increases in aminotransferase levels occur in about one-third of patients; levels usually return to normal even when treatment is continued, but symptomatic retinoid hepatitis can occur and rarely progresses to cirrhosis. Decreases in HDL cholesterol, hypertriglyceridemia, skeletal hyperostosis,

Usual Adult Dosage[1]	Cost[2]
210 mg SC at weeks 0, 1, and 2, then q2 weeks	$10,500.00
160 mg SC at week 0, then 80 mg at weeks 2, 4, 6, 8, 10, and 12, then 80 mg q4 weeks	16,104.00
300 mg[17] SC at weeks 0, 1, 2, 3, and 4, then q4 weeks	15,534.00[18]
100 mg SC at weeks 0 and 4, then q8 weeks	21,718.90[12]
150 mg SC at weeks 0 and 4, then q12 weeks	14,750.00
100 mg SC at weeks 0 and 4, then q12 weeks[19]	13,256.00

18. A carton containing a 300-mg dose (two 150 mg/mL pens or syringes) costs the same as a carton containing a 150-mg dose (one 150 mg/mL pen or syringe).
19. The labeling recommends that tildrakizumab be administered by a healthcare professional.

conjunctivitis, corneal erosions and opacities, iritis, and decreased visual acuity can also occur.

Drug Interactions – Concurrent use of alcohol and acitretin can lead to formation of etretinate, a teratogenic retinoid that has a longer elimination half-life than acitretin; women of childbearing potential should not consume alcohol while taking acitretin and for 2 months after stopping the drug. Acitretin decreases the efficacy of oral progestin-only contraceptives (mini-pills); these contraceptives are not recommended for use in women taking acitretin. Concurrent use of acitretin and methotrexate can increase the risk of hepatotoxicity and is contraindicated. Concurrent use of acitretin and tetracyclines can increase intracranial pressure and the risk of pseudotumor cerebri and is contraindicated. Coadministration of acitretin and supplements containing vitamin A can increase the risk of vitamin A toxicity.

Pregnancy and Lactation – Acitretin is a long-lasting teratogen; patients should not become pregnant or donate blood while taking the drug and for at least 3 years after stopping it. Acitretin is secreted into human breast milk and should not be used in women who are breastfeeding.

APREMILAST — The phosphodiesterase 4 inhibitor apremilast *(Otezla)* is FDA-approved for oral treatment of moderate to severe plaque psoriasis in adults. In 2 randomized, double-blind trials in a total of 1257 patients, significantly more patients achieved a PASI 75 response after 16 weeks with apremilast than with placebo (33% and 29% vs 5% and 6%).[17,18] In an extension study, 45.9% of patients who continued taking apremilast maintained a response after 2 years of treatment.[19]

Adverse Effects – The most common adverse effects of apremilast in clinical trials were diarrhea, nausea, upper respiratory infection, and headache. These effects occurred most frequently during the first 2 weeks of treatment and tended to resolve with continued use of the drug; initial titration of the dose can improve tolerability. Apremilast can increase the risk of depression. Loss of 5-10% of body weight has been reported.

Drug Interactions – Apremilast is metabolized primarily by CYP3A4; concomitant use of apremilast with strong CYP enzyme inducers such as rifampin or carbamazepine can reduce the efficacy of apremilast and is not recommended.[16]

Pregnancy and Lactation – There are no adequate studies of apremilast use in pregnant women. Spontaneous abortions, skeletal abnormalities, dystocia, and reduced birth weights have been reported in animals given apremilast at doses higher than the recommended human dose. Apremilast has been detected in the milk of lactating mice. There are no data on the presence of apremilast in human breast milk or its effects on the breastfed infant or milk production.

BIOLOGIC AGENTS

Updated guidelines for treatment of psoriasis with biologic agents have recently been published.[20] Biologic agents appear to be the most effective treatment for moderate to severe psoriasis, but they may lose efficacy over time and data from head-to-head trials with careful dosage adjustments are limited.[11,21] In patients who have an inadequate response to monotherapy, combining a biologic agent with phototherapy or traditional systemic therapy may improve outcomes, but data are limited and the long-term safety of such combinations is unknown. Switching from one biologic agent to another when the response to the first one is inadequate has been effective in some patients.

TNF INHIBITORS — Four TNF inhibitors, **etanercept** (*Enbrel*, and biosimiliars), **infliximab** (*Remicade*, and biosimilars)*,* **adalimumab** (*Humira*, and biosimiliars), and **certolizumab pegol** *(Cimzia)*, are FDA-approved for treatment of moderate to severe plaque psoriasis. In one review of randomized, double-blind trials comparing their efficacy for this indication, PASI 75 response rates with infliximab, adalimumab, and etanercept within a 12-week period were 78.6%, 70.5%, and 48.1%, respectively.[22] In two randomized trials, PASI 75 response rates with certolizumab pegol were 66.5% and 81.4% compared to 6.5% and 11.6% with placebo.[23] Use of methotrexate in combination with TNF inhibitors may improve efficacy and reduce the risk of anti-drug antibody formation.[20]

Adverse Effects – Serious infections, including bacterial infections (particularly pneumonia and cellulitis), histoplasmosis, and reactivation of hepatitis B virus and tuberculosis (TB), have been reported with all of the TNF inhibitors, particularly during the first 2-7 months of treatment.[24] These drugs should not be given to patients with active localized or chronic infections. Patients should be screened for TB before starting anti-TNF therapy and annually thereafter. Lymphoma and other malignancies have been reported in patients with rheumatoid arthritis receiving a TNF inhibitor, but a causal relationship has not been established. TNF inhibitors generally should not be used in patients with a recent malignancy. Exacerbations and new onset of heart failure, pancytopenia, and demyelinating disorders such as multiple sclerosis have been reported.[25] Anti-TNF drugs have been associated with development of auto-antibodies and induction of a lupus-like syndrome. A review of clinical studies found that anti-drug antibodies reduced the efficacy of infliximab and adalimumab, but not of etanercept.[26]

IL-12/23 ANTAGONIST — Ustekinumab *(Stelara)*, a human monoclonal antibody directed against the p40 subunit shared by interleukin (IL)-12 and -23 cytokines, is FDA-approved for treatment of moderate to severe plaque psoriasis.[27] In a randomized, double-blind trial, PASI 75 responses occurred in 66.7% of patients who received ustekinumab 45 mg and in 75.7% of those who received ustekinumab 90 mg, compared to 3.7% who received placebo.[28] In another randomized trial, ustekinumab was more effective than etanercept (PASI 75 response rates with ustekinumab 45 mg and 90 mg were 67.5% and 73.8%, respectively, vs 56.8% with etanercept).[29]

Adverse Effects – The most common adverse effects of ustekinumab reported during clinical trials in patients with psoriasis were nasopharyngitis, upper respiratory infection, and headache. Ustekinumab has been associated with serious infections (including TB) and malignancies, but long-term safety evaluations have found no increased risk.[30] Patients should be screened for TB before starting treatment. Hypersensitivity reactions (including pneumonitis) and (in one patient) reversible posterior leukoencephalopathy have been reported. Anti-drug antibodies have developed; they may reduce the efficacy of ustekinumab.

IL-17A ANTAGONISTS — Three IL-17A antagonists, secukinumab *(Cosentyx)*, **ixekizumab** *(Taltz)*, and **brodalumab** *(Siliq)*, are FDA-approved for treatment of moderate to severe plaque psoriasis in adults. Secukinumab, a human IgG1 antibody, and ixekizumab, a humanized IgG4 antibody, target IL-17A. Brodalumab, a human IgG2 antibody, binds to the IL-17A receptor. There are no head-to-head comparisons of these 3 agents for this indication, but their PASI 75 response rates have been similar: 77-87% with secukinumab; 87-89% with ixekizumab; and 83-86% with brodalumab.[31-33] In clinical trials, secukinumab and ixekizumab were more effective than etanercept and all 3 IL-17A antagonists were more effective than ustekinumab.[34-38]

Adverse Effects – IL-17A antagonists have been associated with an increased risk of mucocutaneous candidiasis.[39,40] More serious infections have also been reported with use of IL-17A antagonists. Patients should be screened for TB before starting treatment. Onset and exacerbations of Crohn's disease and ulcerative colitis have been reported with these agents.

Neutralizing antibodies have developed in patients treated with secukinumab, but do not appear to be associated with loss of efficacy. Formation of neutralizing antibodies associated with loss of effectiveness has been reported with ixekizumab and brodalumab.

The most common adverse effects of **secukinumab** in clinical trials were nasopharyngitis, diarrhea, and upper respiratory infection. The most common adverse effects of **ixekizumab** were nasopharyngitis, upper respiratory infection, and injection-site reactions, which occurred in 10-15% of patients. Common adverse effects of **brodalumab** included arthralgia, headache, fatigue, diarrhea, oropharyngeal pain, nausea, myalgia, injection-site reactions, influenza, neutropenia, and tinea infections. Suicidal ideation and behavior, including four completed suicides, occurred during clinical trials of brodalumab in patients with plaque psoriasis. Because of this risk, brodalumab is only available through a Risk Evaluation Mitigation Strategy (REMS) program. No association between use of ixekizumab or secukinumab and suicidal behavior has been reported to date.[41]

IL-23 ANTAGONISTS — Guselkumab *(Tremfya)*, a human IgG1 antibody, **tildrakizumab** *(Ilumya)* and **risankizumab** *(Skyrizi)*, both humanized monoclonal IgG1 antibodies, are FDA-approved for treatment of moderate to severe plaque psoriasis in adults. They selectively bind to the p19 subunit of IL-23, inhibiting it from binding to the IL-23 receptor and preventing downstream release of pro-inflammatory cytokines (such as IL-17A) and chemokines.[42-44]

Guselkumab has been more effective than placebo, ustekinumab, or adalimumab in randomized, double-blind trials. In one trial, after 16 weeks, significantly more patients had achieved a PASI 90 response with guselkumab (73.3%) than with adalimumab (49.7%) or placebo (2.9%).[45] In another trial in patients whose psoriasis had not adequately responded to ustekinumab, switching to guselkumab was significantly more effective than continuing ustekinumab.[46] Guselkumab has also been effective in patients who did not respond to adalimumab.[47]

In 2 double-blind, randomized trials, significantly more patients achieved a PASI 75 response after 12 weeks with **tildrakizumab** than with placebo (64% and 61% vs 6%) or etanercept (61% vs 48%).[48]

In clinical trials, **risankizumab** has been more effective than placebo, ustekinumab, or adalimumab. In 2 randomized, double-blind trials, significantly more patients achieved a PASI 90 response after 16 weeks with risankizumab (75.3% and 74.8%) than with placebo (4.9% and 2%) or ustekinumab (42.0% and 47.5%).[49] In another trial, significantly more patients achieved a PASI 90 response after 16 weeks with risankizumab than with adalimumab (72.4% vs 47.4%). In patients who initially had an intermediate response (PASI 50-<90) to adalimumab after 16 weeks, switching to risankizumab was more effective than continuing adalimumab.[50]

Adverse Effects – The most common adverse effects of **guselkumab** have included tinea infections, herpes simplex infections, and gastroenteritis. Serious hypersensitivity reactions and serious infections, including deep fungal infections, have occurred in patients treated with the drug. Antibody formation has been reported with use of guselkumab; whether it reduces the effectiveness of the drug is unknown.

In clinical trials, the most common adverse effects of **tildrakizumab** were upper respiratory infection, injection-site reactions, and diarrhea. Hypersensitivity reactions (angioedema and urticaria) occurred rarely. Neutralizing antibodies developed in 2.5% of patients treated with tildrakizumab for up to 64 weeks; whether they reduce the drug's effectiveness is unknown.

The most common adverse effects reported with **risankizumab** were upper respiratory infection, fatigue, injection-site reactions, and tinea infections. By week 52, neutralizing antibodies had developed in 14% of patients treated with risankizumab; in some patients, high antibody titers were associated with low drug concentrations and reduced clinical response.

Patients should be screened for TB before starting an IL-23 antagonist.

DRUG INTERACTIONS — Patients being treated with **biologic agents** should not receive live vaccines. Proinflammatory cytokines can alter the formation of CYP enzymes. Starting treatment with an inhibitor of TNF, IL-17A, IL-12, or IL-23 may normalize CYP enzyme formation and could alter metabolism of CYP substrates; dosage adjustments of substrates with narrow therapeutic indices such as warfarin or cyclosporine may be needed. **Ustekinumab** may decrease the protective effect of allergen immunotherapy.

PREGNANCY AND LACTATION — **TNF inhibitors** are generally considered safe for use during pregnancy. Placental transfer of anti-TNF antibodies is higher in the late second trimester and in the third trimester, especially with infliximab and adalimumab. Placental transfer is minimal with certolizumab pegol. Human IgG antibodies cross the placenta (especially in the third trimester). There are no adequate data on the use of **ustekinumab**, **IL-17A antagonists**, or **IL-23 antagonists** in pregnant women.[1]

TNF inhibitors are generally considered safe for use in women who are breastfeeding; serum concentrations of TNF inhibitors in human breast milk are expected to be minimal.[8] **Ustekinumab** has been detected in the milk of lactating monkeys. No data are available on the presence of **ustekinumab**, **IL-17A antagonists**, or **IL-23 antagonists** in human breast milk or their effects on the breastfed infant or milk production.

1. MB Hoffman et al. Psoriasis during pregnancy: characteristics and important management recommendations. Expert Rev Clin Immunol 2015; 11:709.
2. Calcipotriene for psoriasis. Med Lett Drugs Ther 1994; 36:70.

3. Calcipotriene/betamethasone foam (Enstilar) for psoriasis. Med Lett Drugs Ther 2016; 58:48.
4. Calcitriol (Vectical) for mild to moderate plaque psoriasis. Med Lett Drugs Ther 2009; 51:70.
5. DM Pariser et al. Halobetasol 0.01%/tazarotene 0.045% lotion in the treatment of moderate-to-severe plaque psoriasis: maintenance of therapeutic effect after cessation of therapy. J Drugs Dermatol 2018; 17:723.
6. A Menter et al. Guidelines of care for the management of psoriasis and psoriatic arthritis. Section 3. Guidelines of care for the management and treatment of psoriasis with topical therapies. J Am Acad Dermatol 2009; 60:643.
7. A Dattola et al. Update of calcineurin inhibitors to treat inverse psoriasis: A systematic review. Dermatol Ther 2018; 31:e12728.
8. DC Butler et al. Safety of dermatologic medications in pregnancy and lactation. Part II: lactation. J Am Acad Dermatol 2014; 70:417.
9. X Chen et al. Narrow-band ultraviolet B phototherapy versus broad-band ultraviolet B or psoralen-ultraviolet A photochemotherapy for psoriasis. Cochrane Database Syst Rev 2013; 10:CD009481.
10. MB Totonchy and MW Chiu. UV-based therapy. Dermatol Clin 2014; 32:399.
11. E Sbidian et al. Systemic pharmacological treatments for chronic plaque psoriasis: a network meta-analysis. Cochrane Database Syst Rev 2017; 12: CD011535.
12. RB Warren et al. An intensified dosing schedule of subcutaneous methotrexate in patients with moderate to severe plaque-type psoriasis (METOP): a 52 week, multicentre, randomised, double-blind, placebo-controlled, phase 3 trial. Lancet 2017; 389:528.
13. ED Dommasch et al. Risk of serious infection in patients receiving systemic medications for the treatment of psoriasis. JAMA Dermatol 2019 May 10 (epub).
14. VM Heydendael et al. Methotrexate versus cyclosporine in moderate-to-severe chronic plaque psoriasis. N Engl J Med 2003; 349:658.
15. I Flytström et al. Methotrexate vs. ciclosporin in psoriasis: effectiveness, quality of life and safety. A randomized controlled trial. Br J Dermatol 2008; 158;116.
16. Inhibitors and inducers of CYP enzymes and P-glycoprotein. Med Lett Drugs Ther 2017 September 18 (epub). Available at: medicalletter.org/downloads/CYP_PGP_Tables.pdf.
17. K Papp et al. Apremilast, an oral phosphodiesterase 4 (PDE4) inhibitor, in patients with moderate to severe plaque psoriasis: results of a phase III, randomized, controlled trial (Efficacy and Safety Trial Evaluating the Effects of Apremilast in Psoriasis [ESTEEM] 1). J Am Acad Dermatol 2015; 73:37.
18. C Paul et al. Efficacy and safety of apremilast, an oral phosphodiesterase 4 inhibitor, in patients with moderate-to-severe plaque psoriasis over 52 weeks: a phase III, randomized controlled trial (ESTEEM 2). Br J Dermatol 2015; 173:1387.
19. K Reich et al. Safety and efficacy of apremilast through 104 weeks in patients with moderate to severe psoriasis who continued on apremilast or switched from etanercept treatment: findings from the LIBERATE study. J Eur Acad Dermatol Venereol 2018; 32:397.
20. A Menter et al. Joint AAD-NPF guidelines of care for the management and treatment of psoriasis with biologics. J Am Acad Dermatol 2019; 80:1029.
21. A Egeberg et al. Safety, efficacy and drug survival of biologics and biosimilars for moderate-to-severe plaque psoriasis. Br J Dermatol 2018; 78:509.

22. IH Kim et al. Comparative efficacy of biologics in psoriasis: a review. Am J Clin Dermatol 2012; 13:365.

23. AB Gottlieb et al. Certolizumab pegol for the treatment of chronic plaque psoriasis: results through 48 weeks from 2 phase 3, multicenter, randomized, double-blinded, placebo-controlled studies (CIMPASI-1 and CIMPASI-2). J Am Acad Dermatol 2018; 79:302.

24. RE Kalb et al. Risk of serious infection with biologic and systemic treatment of psoriasis: results from the psoriasis longitudinal assessment and registry (PSOLAR). JAMA Dermatol 2015; 151:961.

25. AL Semble et al. Safety and tolerability of tumor necrosis factor-α inhibitors in psoriasis: a narrative review. Am J Clin Dermatol 2014; 15:37.

26. L Hsu et al. Antidrug antibodies in psoriasis: a systematic review. Br J Dermatol 2014; 170:261.

27. Ustekinumab (Stelara) for psoriasis. Med Lett Drugs Ther 2010; 52:7.

28. KA Papp et al. Efficacy and safety of ustekinumab, a human interleukin-12/23 monoclonal antibody, in patients with psoriasis: 52-week results from a randomised, double-blind, placebo-controlled trial (PHOENIX 2). Lancet 2008; 371:1675.

29. CE Griffiths et al. Comparison of ustekinumab and etanercept for moderate-to-severe psoriasis. N Engl J Med 2010; 362:118.

30. KA Papp et al. Long-term safety of ustekinumab in patients with moderate-to-severe psoriasis: final results from 5 years of follow-up. Br J Dermatol 2013; 168:844.

31. Secukinumab (Cosentyx) for psoriasis. Med Lett Drugs Ther 2015; 57:45.

32. Ixekizumab (Taltz) – a second IL-17A inhibitor for psoriasis. Med Lett Drugs Ther 2016; 58:59.

33. Brodalumab (Siliq) – another IL-17A antagonist for psoriasis. Med Lett Drugs Ther 2017; 59:118.

34. M Lebwohl et al. Phase 3 studies comparing brodalumab with ustekinumab in psoriasis. N Engl J Med 2015; 373:1318.

35. J Bagel et al. Secukinumab is superior to ustekinumab in clearing skin in patients with moderate to severe plaque psoriasis (16-week CLARITY results). Dermatol Ther (Heidelb) 2018; 8:571.

36. K Reich et al. Comparison of ixekizumab with ustekinumab in moderate-to-severe psoriasis: 24-week results from IXORA-S, a phase III study. Br J Dermatol 2017; 177:1014.

37. RG Langley et al. Secukinumab in plaque psoriasis – results of two phase 3 trials. N Engl J Med 2014; 371:326.

38. CE Griffiths et al. Comparison of ixekizumab with etanercept or placebo in moderate-to-severe psoriasis (UNCOVER-2 and UNCOVER-3): results from two phase 3 randomised trials. Lancet 2015; 386:541.

39. A Deodhar et al. Long-term safety of secukinumab in patients with moderate-to-severe plaque psoriasis, psoriatic arthritis, and ankylosing spondylitis: integrated pooled clinical trial and post-marketing surveillance data. Arthritis Res Ther 2019; 21:111.

40. KA Papp et al. Infections from seven clinical trials of ixekizumab, an anti-interleukin-17A monoclonal antibody, in patients with moderate-to-severe psoriasis. Br J Dermatol 2017; 177:1537.

41. A Chiricozzi et al. No meaningful association between suicidal behavior and the use of IL-17A-neutralizing or IL-17RA-blocking agents. Expert Opin Drug Saf 2016; 15:1653.

42. Guselkumab (Tremfya) for psoriasis. Med Lett Drugs Ther. 2017; 59:179.

43. Tildrakizumab (Ilumya) – another IL-23 antagonist for psoriasis. Med Lett Drugs Ther 2019; 61:4.

44. Risankizumab (Skyrizi) – a new IL-23 antagonist for plaque psoriasis. Med Lett Drugs Ther 2019; 61:81.

45. A Blauvelt et al. Efficacy and safety of guselkumab, an anti-interleukin-23 monoclonal antibody, compared with adalimumab for the continuous treatment of patients with moderate to severe psoriasis: results from the phase III, double-blinded, placebo- and active comparator-controlled VOYAGE 1 trial. J Am Acad Dermatol 2017; 76:405.

46. RG Langley et al. Efficacy and safety of guselkumab in patients with psoriasis who have an inadequate response to ustekinumab: results of the randomized, double-blind, phase III NAVIGATE trial. Br J Dermatol 2018; 178:114.

47. K Reich et al. Efficacy and safety of guselkumab, an anti-interleukin-23 monoclonal antibody, compared with adalimumab for the treatment of patients with moderate to severe psoriasis with randomized withdrawal and retreatment: results from the phase III, double-blind, placebo- and active comparator-controlled VOYAGE 2 trial. J Am Acad Dermatol 2017; 76:418.

48. K Reich et al. Tildrakizumab versus placebo or etanercept for chronic plaque psoriasis (reSURFACE 1 and reSURFACE 2): results from two randomised controlled, phase 3 trials. Lancet 2017; 390:276.

49. KB Gordon et al. Efficacy and safety of risankizumab in moderate-to-severe plaque psoriasis (UltIMMa-1 and UltIMMa-2): results from two double-blind, randomised, placebo-controlled and ustekinumab-controlled phase 3 trials. Lancet 2018; 392:650.

50. K Reich et al. Efficacy and safety of continuous risankizumab or switching from adalimumab to risankizumab treatment in patients with moderate-to-severe plaque psoriasis: results from the phase 3 IMMvent trial. American Academy of Dermatology Annual Meeting, Washington, DC, March 1-5, 2019. Poster 10218.

DRUGS FOR
Psoriatic Arthritis

Original publication date – December 2019

Psoriatic arthritis is a chronic inflammatory arthropathy associated with psoriasis. A recent review found that about 20% of patients with psoriasis have psoriatic arthritis.[1] Updated guidelines for treatment of psoriatic arthritis have recently been published.[2]

SYMPTOMATIC TREATMENT

NSAIDs — Nonsteroidal anti-inflammatory drugs (NSAIDs) can improve symptoms in patients with psoriatic arthritis. They can be used as monotherapy in those with mild disease.

Dyspepsia and GI ulceration, perforation, and bleeding can occur with NSAID use. Nonselective NSAIDs can interfere with platelet function and prolong bleeding time. The COX-2 selective NSAID celecoxib (*Celebrex*, and generics) does not affect platelets significantly and is less likely than nonselective NSAIDs to cause GI toxicity, but it may have a prothrombotic effect.[3] All NSAIDs inhibit renal prostaglandins, decrease renal blood flow, cause fluid retention, and may cause hypertension and renal failure in some patients.

CORTICOSTEROIDS — When only a few joints are involved, intra-articular injections of corticosteroids may provide symptomatic relief. Low doses of systemic corticosteroids (5-10 mg/day) have also

Summary: Treatment of Psoriatic Arthritis

- ► NSAIDs can relieve joint symptoms and can be used as monotherapy in patients with mild disease.
- ► When only a few joints are involved, intra-articular injection of a corticosteroid can provide relief of arthritis symptoms. Low doses of systemic corticosteroids may also be used short-term for symptom relief.
- ► Conventional DMARDs can be used for first-line treatment of mild to moderate psoriatic arthritis; methotrexate, leflunomide (*Arava*, and generics), and sulfasalazine (*Azulfidine*, and generics) are the most widely used conventional DMARDs.
- ► Apremilast (*Otezla*) has been safe and modestly effective; it could be considered as an alternative to DMARDs in patients with mild to moderate psoriatic arthritis, but it has not been shown to slow joint damage and it is expensive.
- ► TNF inhibitors are recommended for first-line treatment of moderate to severe psoriatic arthritis. They are preferred for patients who have had an inadequate response to conventional DMARDs. Patients who do not respond to one TNF inhibitor may respond to another.
- ► The IL-12 and -23 inhibitor ustekinumab (*Stelara*) or the IL-17A inhibitors secukinumab (*Cosentyx*) and ixekizumab (*Taltz*) can be used in patients who have not responded to one or more TNF inhibitors.
- ► The T-cell costimulation modulator abatacept (*Orencia*) is an option for patients who have not responded to other biologics.
- ► The JAK inhibitor tofacitinib (*Xeljanz*) may be considered for patients who have not responded to conventional DMARDs or a TNF inhibitor and prefer oral therapy.
- ► Biologics/JAK inhibitors may be used in combination with conventional DMARDs, but they should not be used with other biologics/JAK inhibitors.

been used short-term for symptom relief. Long-term use of systemic corticosteroids can increase the risk of infection and cause fluid retention, osteoporosis, osteonecrosis, cataracts, glaucoma, impaired skin healing, acne, insomnia, mood disorders, Cushing's syndrome, hyperglycemia, and adrenal suppression and is not recommended.

CONVENTIONAL DMARDs

Conventional (non-biologic) disease-modifying antirheumatic drugs (DMARDs) can be used for treatment of mild to moderate disease or for treatment of moderate to severe disease in patients who are unable to use TNF inhibitors or prefer oral therapy. They have not been shown to prevent progression of joint damage in patients with psoriatic arthritis.

METHOTREXATE — Methotrexate (*Trexall*, and others) is probably the most widely used conventional DMARD for treatment of psoriasis and psoriatic arthritis (it is not FDA-approved for use in psoriatic arthritis). Observational studies have reported beneficial clinical effects, but evidence from controlled trials is limited.[4] In one randomized, double-blind trial in 851 patients with active psoriatic arthritis who were naive to biologic treatment and had not previously used methotrexate for this disorder, 51% of patients who received methotrexate monotherapy (target 20 mg/week) achieved an ACR20 response (20% improvement on the American College of Rheumatology scale) at week 24 compared to 61% of those who received etanercept monotherapy and 65% of patients treated with the combination of methotrexate and etanercept.[5]

Adverse Effects – In the doses recommended for psoriatic arthritis, methotrexate is usually well tolerated, but it can cause stomatitis, anorexia, nausea, vomiting, abdominal cramps, fatigue, aminotransferase elevations, and hepatic fibrosis. GI adverse effects associated with oral methotrexate are less likely to occur with parenteral administration. Hepatotoxicity is the most frequent serious adverse effect; the drug is contraindicated for use in patients with alcohol use disorder. Methotrexate is immunosuppressive and should not be used in patients with an active infection. Methotrexate-induced pneumonitis is rare, but can be fatal. Macrocytic anemia, leukopenia, and thrombocytopenia can occur. Liver function and blood counts should be monitored. Decreased renal function and inadvertent overdosing (daily rather than weekly) are common causes of hematologic toxicity.

Drug Interactions – Trimethoprim and other drugs that interfere with folate metabolism may increase bone marrow suppression caused by methotrexate. Proton pump inhibitors (PPIs) and drugs that reduce renal function, particularly NSAIDs, may increase serum concentrations of methotrexate and possibly its toxicity. Concurrent use of methotrexate and alcohol or hepatotoxic drugs, such as acitretin (*Soriatane*, and generics), may increase the risk of hepatotoxicity.

Pregnancy and Lactation – Methotrexate is teratogenic and abortifacient and is contraindicated for use during pregnancy; after stopping it, men should wait a minimum of 3 months and women should probably wait as long as 6 months before attempting to conceive.[6] Methotrexate has been detected in human breast milk; it is contraindicated for use in breastfeeding women.

LEFLUNOMIDE — An oral inhibitor of pyrimidine synthesis, leflunomide (*Arava*, and generics) is often used for treatment of psoriatic arthritis in patients who have not responded to methotrexate or cannot tolerate it. In a randomized, double-blind, 24-week trial in 190 patients, the psoriatic arthritis response criteria (PsARC) response rate was 59% with leflunomide and 30% with placebo.[7]

Adverse Effects – Leflunomide is immunosuppressive. Diarrhea occurs frequently. Reversible alopecia, rash, hypertension, myelosuppression, and aminotransferase elevations have also been reported. Anaphylaxis, Stevens-Johnson syndrome, weight loss, interstitial lung disease, peripheral neuropathy, and leukocytoclastic vasculitis have occurred rarely. If severe toxicity occurs and leflunomide must be discontinued, cholestyramine (*Questran*, and others) should be used to bind and eliminate the drug; without cholestyramine, it could take up to 2 years for serum concentrations of the drug to become undetectable.

Drug Interactions – Leflunomide is metabolized *in vitro* by CYP1A2, 2C19, and 3A4. Concurrent use of rifampin, a CYP inducer, and leflunomide can increase serum concentrations of teriflunomide, the active metabolite of leflunomide; caution should be used if these drugs are coadministered. Teriflunomide can decrease the INR in patients who are taking warfarin. Use of leflunomide with oral contraceptives can increase serum concentrations of ethinyl estradiol and levonorgestrel. Teriflunomide is an inhibitor of CYP2C8 and the drug transporters organic anion transporter

(OAT) 3, breast cancer resistance protein (BCRP), and organic anion transporting polypeptide (OATP) 1B1 and 1B3; use of leflunomide with substrates of CYP2C8, OAT3, BCRP, or OATP1B1/3 can increase their serum concentrations.

Pregnancy and Lactation – Animal studies indicate that leflunomide taken during pregnancy may have teratogenic effects or increase the risk of fetal death. The drug is contraindicated for use during pregnancy. It should be stopped before conception, and women should take cholestyramine to bind and eliminate the drug; without cholestyramine, it could take up to 2 years for serum concentrations of the drug to become undetectable. No data are available on the presence of leflunomide in human breast milk or its effects on the breastfed infant or milk production; because of the potential for serious adverse reactions, women taking leflunomide should not breastfeed.

SULFASALAZINE — In clinical trials, sulfasalazine (*Azulfidine*, and generics) has produced modest improvements in psoriatic arthritis symptoms.[8]

Adverse Effects – Sulfasalazine frequently causes GI disturbances. Leukopenia, agranulocytosis, reversible oligospermia, a lupus-like syndrome, and hepatotoxicity have been reported.

Drug Interactions – Sulfasalazine may decrease serum concentrations of digoxin (*Lanoxin*, and others). It inhibits thiopurine methyltransferase (TPMT) and may decrease the metabolism of azathioprine (*Imuran*, and others) and 6-MP, which could increase their toxicity, especially in patients with inherited TPMT deficiency.

Pregnancy and Lactation – Sulfasalazine is generally considered safe for use during pregnancy, but neural tube defects have been reported in infants born to women who took it during pregnancy. The drug inhibits the absorption and metabolism of folic acid; pregnant women taking sulfasalazine may need higher doses of folic acid. Sulfasalazine is secreted into human breast milk in small amounts and is considered safe

Table 1. Some Systemic Drugs for Psoriatic Arthritis

Drug	Usual Adult Dosage[1]	Cost[2]
Conventional DMARDs		
Cyclosporine[3] – generic	2.5-4 mg/kg/day PO in 2 divided doses	$1582.70
Neoral (Novartis)		3072.00
Gengraf (Abbvie)		2518.70
Leflunomide[3] – generic	10-20 mg PO once/day	501.90
Arava (Sanofi)		7376.50
Methotrexate, oral[3] – generic	7.5-25 mg/week PO in a single dose or in 3 divided doses over 36 hours	164.60
Methotrexate, injectable[3] – generic	10-25 mg SC or IM once/week	17.50
Otrexup[4] (Antares)	10-25 mg SC once/week	3898.80
Rasuvo[4] (Medac)	10-25 mg SC once/week	2958.00
RediTrex[4] (Cumberland)	10-25 mg SC once/week	N.A.
Sulfasalazine[3] – generic	2-3 g/day PO in divided doses	133.90
Azulfidine (Pfizer)		1087.00
enteric-coated – generic		191.20
Azulfidine EN-tabs		1419.70
Phosphodiesterase Type-4 Inhibitor		
Apremilast – *Otezla* (Celgene)	30 mg PO bid[5]	20,388.00

N.A. = not yet available
1. Dosage adjustments may be needed for renal or hepatic impairment.
2. Approximate WAC for 24 weeks' treatment at the lowest usual adult maintenance dosage (cost of initial doses are not included). Cyclosporine, infliximab, and *Simponi Aria* cost calculated for a patient weighing 80 kg. WAC = wholesaler acquisition cost or manufacturer's published price to wholesalers; WAC represents a published catalogue or list price and may not represent an actual transactional price. Source: AnalySource® Monthly. December 5, 2019. Reprinted with permission by First Databank, Inc. All rights reserved. ©2019. www.fdbhealth.com/policies/drug-pricing-policy.
3. Not FDA-approved for treatment of psoriatic arthritis.
4. *Otrexup* and *Rasuvo* are available as single-dose auto-injectors. *RediTrex* is available as single-dose pre-filled syringes.
5. The recommended starting dose is 10 mg once daily, which should be titrated over 5 days to the maintenance dosage of 30 mg twice daily to reduce the risk of GI adverse effects. The dosage should be reduced to 30 mg once/day in patients with severe renal impairment (CrCl <30 mL/min).

Continued on next page

Table 1. Some Systemic Drugs for Psoriatic Arthritis (continued)

Drug	Usual Adult Dosage[1]	Cost[2]
TNF Inhibitors		
Adalimumab – *Humira* (Abbvie)[6,7]	40 mg SC q2 weeks[8]	$31,044.50
Certolizumab pegol – *Cimzia* (UCB)	400 mg SC at 0, 2, and 4 weeks, then 200 mg q2 weeks or 400 mg q4 weeks[8]	25,964.60
Etanercept – *Enbrel* (Amgen)[9]	50 mg SC once/week[8]	31,044.50
Golimumab – *Simponi* (Janssen)	50 mg SC once/month	28,854.10
Simponi Aria	2 mg/kg IV at 0 and 4 weeks, then q8 weeks	21,822.10
Infliximab – *Remicade* (Janssen) biosimilars[11]	5 mg/kg IV at 0, 2, and 6 weeks, then q8 weeks[10]	14,013.80
Infliximab-abda – *Renflexis* (Merck)		9040.70
Infliximab-dyyb – *Inflectra* (Pfizer)		11,355.40
IL-12 and -23 Inhibitor		
Ustekinumab – *Stelara* (Janssen)	45 mg SC at 0 and 4 weeks, then q12 weeks[8]	22,004.60
IL-17A Inhibitors		
Ixekizumab – *Taltz* (Lilly)	160 mg SC at week 0, then 80 mg q4 weeks[8]	32,208.00

6. Five adalimumab biosimilars (*Abrilada, Amjevita, Cyltezo, Hadlima*, and *Hyrimoz*) have been approved by the FDA, but are not yet available.
7. *Humira Citrate-free* does not contain citrate buffers, which have been associated with injection-site pain (P Nash et al. Rheumatol Ther 2016; 3:257). Compared to original *Humira*, it has a smaller needle and smaller injection volume.
8. Dosage is different for treatment of moderate to severe plaque psoriasis. In patients with both psoriatic arthritis and psoriasis, the psoriasis dosage should be used. Drugs and dosages for treatment of psoriasis can be found here: https://secure.medicalletter.org/TML-article-1574a.
9. *Erelzi* and *Eticovo*, etanercept biosimilars, have been approved by the FDA, but are not yet available.
10. Some patients may require more frequent dosing (every 4 or 6 weeks) and/or a higher dose (10 mg/kg) for adequate disease control.
11. Two other infliximab biosimilars (*Ixifi, Avsola*) have also been approved by the FDA, but are not yet available.

Continued on next page

Table 1. Some Systemic Drugs for Psoriatic Arthritis (continued)

Drug	Usual Adult Dosage[1]	Cost[2]
IL-17A Inhibitors (continued)		
Secukinumab – *Cosentyx* (Novartis)	150 mg SC at 0, 1, 2, 3, and 4 weeks, then q4 weeks or 150 mg q4 weeks[8,12]	$31,073.50[13]
T-Cell Costimulation Modulator		
Abatacept – *Orencia* (BMS)	125 mg SC once/week or 500-1000 mg[14] IV at 0, 2, and 4 weeks, then q4 weeks	26,273.30[15]
Janus Kinase (JAK) Inhibitor		
Tofacitinib – *Xeljanz* (Pfizer)	5 mg PO bid[16]	26,883.80
Xeljanz XR	11 mg PO once/day[16]	26,883.80

12. Consider increasing the dose to 300 mg in patients who continue to have active disease.
13. A carton containing a 300-mg dose (two 150 mg/mL pens or syringes) costs the same as a carton containing a 150-mg dose (one 150 mg/mL pen or syringe).
14. The IV dose is 500 mg for patients weighing <60 kg, 750 mg for those weighing 60-100 kg, and 1000 mg for those weighing >100 kg.
15. Cost for subcutaneous dosage.
16. The dosage should be reduced to 5 mg once daily for patients with moderate to severe renal impairment or moderate hepatic impairment, or for those taking a strong CYP3A4 inhibitor or a moderate CYP3A4 inhibitor with a strong CYP2C19 inhibitor. The dosage may also need to be reduced for patients with lymphopenia, neutropenia, or anemia.

for use in most breastfeeding women, but because of an increased risk of hemolysis, women taking sulfasalazine should not breastfeed premature infants or infants with hyperbilirubinemia or glucose 6-phosphate dehydrogenase (G6PD) deficiency.

CYCLOSPORINE — Use of cyclosporine (*Neoral*, and others) in patients with psoriatic arthritis has resulted in modest improvements in pain and other symptoms in small, open-label studies.[9] In a 12-month, randomized, double-blind, placebo-controlled trial in 72 patients with an incomplete response to methotrexate, addition of cyclosporine significantly reduced signs of joint inflammation, but did not improve pain or quality of life.[10] Use of cyclosporine has been limited by the risk of nephrotoxicity.[11]

Adverse Effects – The doses of cyclosporine used for treatment of psoriatic arthritis are generally safe, but hypertension and nephrotoxicity can occur. Cyclosporine can also cause diarrhea, nausea, vomiting, infection, hirsutism, gingival hyperplasia, pruritus, headache, paresthesias, and hypertriglyceridemia. Hyperuricemia and gout are common with long-term use. The drug also increases the risk of skin malignancies in patients previously treated with psoralens plus UVA radiation (PUVA).

Drug Interactions – Use of cyclosporine with other nephrotoxic drugs such as aminoglycosides can result in additive nephrotoxic effects. Use with potassium-sparing diuretics such as spironolactone (*Aldactone*, and generics) may increase the risk of hyperkalemia. Cyclosporine is both a substrate and an inhibitor of CYP3A4 and P-glycoprotein (P-gp); use with CYP3A4 inhibitors may increase its toxicity and use with CYP3A4 inducers may decrease its effectiveness.[12]

Pregnancy and Lactation – Cyclosporine appears to be relatively safe for use during pregnancy, but it has been associated with low birth weight and premature birth.[13] It is present in human breast milk and detectable levels have been reported in breastfed infants whose mothers were taking the drug.

PDE4 INHIBITOR

APREMILAST — The oral phosphodiesterase type-4 (PDE4) inhibitor apremilast *(Otezla)* is FDA-approved for treatment of active psoriatic arthritis and moderate to severe plaque psoriasis in adults.[14] In randomized, double-blind trials in patients with active psoriatic arthritis despite treatment with conventional or biologic DMARDs, ACR20 response rates after 16 weeks were 32-41% with apremilast compared to 18-19% with placebo; the response of patients in these trials was about the same whether or not they had continued taking their baseline conventional DMARD therapy.[15-17] In an open-label extension trial, after 5 years, 67% of patients who had continued on apremilast had achieved an ACR20 response.[18] Apremilast has also been effective in patients who have not received prior treatment with conventional or biologic DMARDs (ACR20 response: 31% vs 16% with placebo and 38% vs 20%).[19,20] No studies directly comparing apremilast with a TNF inhibitor are available; in cross-study comparisons, response rates appear to be lower with apremilast, and there is no current evidence that it slows joint damage.

Adverse Effects – The most common adverse effects of apremilast in clinical trials were diarrhea, nausea, and headache. These effects occurred most frequently during the first two weeks of treatment and tended to resolve with continued use of the drug. No increased risk of malignancy or serious infection, including reactivation of tuberculosis (TB), has been reported to date. Apremilast can increase the risk of depression. Loss of 5-10% of body weight has been reported.

Drug Interactions – Apremilast is metabolized primarily by CYP3A4. Concomitant use of apremilast with strong CYP enzyme inducers such as rifampin or carbamazepine can reduce the efficacy of apremilast and is not recommended.[12]

Pregnancy and Lactation – There are no adequate studies of apremilast in pregnant women. Spontaneous abortions, skeletal abnormalities, dystocia, and reduced birth weights have been reported in animals given apremilast at doses higher than the recommended human dose. Apremilast has been detected in the milk of lactating mice. There are no data on the presence of apremilast in human breast milk or its effects on the breastfed infant or milk production.

BIOLOGIC DMARDs

TNF INHIBITORS — Five tumor necrosis factor (TNF) inhibitors, **adalimumab** (*Humira*, and biosimilars), **certolizumab pegol** *(Cimzia)*, **etanercept** (*Enbrel*, and biosimilars), **golimumab** *(Simponi)*, and **infliximab** (*Remicade*, and biosimilars), are approved by the FDA for treatment of active psoriatic arthritis; all except golimumab are also approved for treatment of psoriasis. TNF inhibitors are recommended for treatment of moderate to severe disease in treatment-naive patients and are preferred for patients who have had an inadequate response to conventional DMARDs.[2] They have been shown to reduce joint disease activity, prevent structural damage, and improve function, and they may have beneficial effects on bone.[21,22] TNF inhibitors have been associated with less radiographic disease progression than methotrexate.[5,23] Some patients who have not responded to one TNF inhibitor have responded to another.[24]

In clinical trials, ACR20 response rates in patients with psoriatic arthritis were 58% with adalimumab, 52%-58% with certolizumab pegol, 59% with etanercept, 58% with infliximab, and 51% with golimumab after 12-14 weeks of treatment.[8,25-27] No head-to-head comparisons of TNF inhibitors for treatment of psoriatic arthritis are available.

Combination Therapy – Whether combining a conventional DMARD with a TNF inhibitor improves response rates in patients with psoriatic arthritis beyond those achieved by treatment with a TNF inhibitor alone is unclear. In clinical trials of TNF inhibitors that allowed concomitant use of methotrexate, the combination did not appear to improve efficacy.[28] In a randomized, double-blind trial, addition of methotrexate to etanercept did not improve the efficacy of etanercept monotherapy.[5]

In another randomized, double-blind trial in 51 treatment-naive patients with early psoriatic arthritis, significantly more patients achieved remission at 22 weeks with concurrent use of methotrexate and golimumab than with methotrexate alone (81% vs 42%).[29] In an open-label extension, in 18 patients who initially achieved remission with golimumab and methotrexate and at 22 weeks switched to methotrexate alone, 10 were still in remission at week 50.[30]

Methotrexate may reduce the formation of antidrug antibodies in patients taking infliximab or adalimumab.[2] Whether this increases the duration of effective TNF inhibitor therapy is unclear.[31-33]

Adverse Effects – Serious infections, including bacterial infections (particularly pneumonitis and cellulitis), histoplasmosis, and reactivation of TB and hepatitis B virus, have been reported with all the TNF inhibitors.[34] These drugs should not be given to patients with active or chronic infections. Screening for exposure to TB is recommended before starting anti-TNF therapy and annually thereafter. Lymphoma and other malignancies have been reported in patients with rheumatoid arthritis receiving these drugs, but a causal relationship has not been established. TNF inhibitors generally should not be used in patients with a recent malignancy. Exacerbations and new onset of heart failure, pancytopenia, and demyelinating disorders such as multiple sclerosis have been reported.[35] Anti-TNF drugs have been associated with development of autoantibodies and the induction of a lupus-like syndrome. Antidrug antibodies have been associated with lower drug concentrations and sometimes with a reduced response.[36]

IL-12/23 INHIBITOR — The human interleukin (IL)-12 and -23 inhibitor **ustekinumab** *(Stelara)* is FDA-approved for treatment of psoriasis and psoriatic arthritis.[25] In a randomized, double-blind trial in 615 patients with active psoriatic arthritis despite treatment with conventional DMARDs or NSAIDs, 42% of patients treated with ustekinumab achieved an ACR20 response at week 24 compared to 23% of those who received placebo.[37] Ustekinumab also slowed radiographic progression compared to placebo.[38]

Adverse Effects – Ustekinumab has been associated with serious infections (including TB), malignancies, hypersensitivity reactions, and reversible posterior leukoencephalopathy. Screening for TB is recommended before starting ustekinumab treatment. Antidrug antibodies have developed; whether they reduce treatment response in patients with psoriatic arthritis remains to be determined.

IL-17A INHIBITORS — Secukinumab *(Cosentyx)*, a human IgG1 antibody, and ixekizumab *(Taltz)*, a humanized IgG4 antibody, both approved earlier for treatment of moderate to severe plaque psoriasis, have also been approved by the FDA for treatment of psoriatic arthritis.

In 3 randomized, double-blind trials, ACR20 response rates were significantly higher in patients treated with **secukinumab** than in those who received placebo (51% vs 15%, 50.0% vs 17.3%, 56% vs 27%).[39-41] Secukinumab also significantly inhibited radiographic progression of disease.[41] It was effective in both TNF inhibitor-naive and TNF inhibitor-experienced patients.

In a randomized, double-blind, placebo- and active-controlled trial in 417 patients who had never been treated with a biologic agent, ACR20 response rates at 24 weeks were 58% with **ixekizumab**, 57% with adalimumab, and 30% with placebo; both ixekizumab and adalimumab inhibited progression of structural damage.[42] In another trial in 363 patients who had failed TNF inhibitor therapy, ACR20 response rates were 53% with ixekizumab versus 20% with placebo.[43] In a 24-week, head-to-head, open-label, blinded-assessor trial in patients with both skin and joint disease and an inadequate response to conventional DMARDs, ixekizumab was superior to adalimumab for simultaneous achievement of an ACR50 and a PASI100 (100% improvement in Psoriasis Area and Severity Index score) response (35% vs 28%). When evaluated separately, ixekizumab was noninferior to adalimumab for ACR50 response (51% vs 47%) and superior for PASI100 response (60% vs 47%).[44]

Adverse Effects – The most common adverse effects of secukinumab and ixekizumab in clinical trials have included injection site reactions, nausea, tinea infections, and upper respiratory infections. These drugs have also been associated with a higher risk of mucocutaneous *Candida* infections. Patients should be screened for TB before starting therapy. Exacerbations of Crohn's disease were reported during clinical trials. Urticaria and anaphylaxis have occurred. Neutralizing antibodies have developed with both secukinumab and ixekizumab.

T-CELL ACTIVATION INHIBITOR — **Abatacept** *(Orencia)*, a genetically engineered fusion protein that interferes with T-cell activation and has been effective in treating rheumatoid arthritis that has not responded to methotrexate or TNF inhibitors, has now been approved by the FDA for the treatment of adults with active psoriatic arthritis. Approval of abatacept for this indication was based on the results of 2 randomized, double-blind trials. In the first trial, patients with an inadequate response to conventional DMARDs or a TNF inhibitor were randomized to receive placebo or various IV doses of abatacept. An ACR20 response occurred in 47.5% of patients who received a 10 mg/kg dose compared to 19.0% of those who received placebo.[45] The second trial included patients who had not responded to ≥1 non-biologic DMARDs and about 60% of patients had prior exposure to a TNF inhibitor; an ACR20 response occurred in 39.4% of patients who received subcutaneous injections of abatacept compared to 22.3% of those who received placebo.[46]

Adverse Effects – The most serious adverse effects associated with use of abatacept have been serious infections, such as pneumonia or sepsis, and malignancies, including lung cancer and lymphoma. Hypertension, headache, dizziness and, rarely, anaphylactoid reactions can occur within one hour after the start of an abatacept infusion. Adverse effects such as COPD exacerbation, rhonchi, and dyspnea occurred more often in COPD patients who were treated with abatacept than in those treated with placebo. In the clinical trials in patients with psoriatic arthritis, the most common adverse effects were nasopharyngitis, upper respiratory tract infections, and bronchitis.

DRUG INTERACTIONS — Use of multiple biologic drugs at the same time can increase the risk of serious infections and is not recommended. Patients being treated with biologic agents should not receive live vaccines. Proinflammatory cytokines can alter the formation of CYP enzymes; starting treatment with a TNF or IL inhibitor may normalize CYP enzyme formation and could alter the metabolism of CYP substrates. Dosage adjustments of substrates with narrow therapeutic indices such as warfarin or cyclosporine may be needed. Ustekinumab may decrease the protective effect of allergen immunotherapy.

PREGNANCY AND LACTATION — TNF inhibitors are generally considered safe for use during pregnancy. Placental transfer of anti-TNF antibodies is higher in the late second trimester and in the third trimester. Placental transfer is minimal with certolizumab pegol. Human IgG antibodies cross the placenta (especially in the third trimester). There are no adequate data on the use of ustekinumab, IL-17A inhibitors, or abatacept in pregnant women.[13]

TNF inhibitors are generally considered safe for use in women who are breastfeeding; serum concentrations of TNF inhibitors in human breast milk are expected to be minimal.[47] No data are available on the presence of ustekinumab, IL-17A antagonists, or abatacept in human breast milk or their effects on the breastfed infant or milk production.

JAK INHIBITORS

TOFACITINIB — Tofacitinib *(Xeljanz, Xeljanz XR)*, a synthetic oral inhibitor of Janus kinase (JAK), is an important signaling mediator in various immune activation pathways.[48] It is FDA-approved for treatment of active psoriatic arthritis in adults who have had an inadequate response or intolerance to methotrexate or other DMARDs. In a randomized, double-blind, placebo- and active-controlled trial in patients with active psoriatic arthritis who had previously had an inadequate response to conventional DMARD therapy, ACR20 response rates were 50% with tofacitinib compared to 52% with adalimumab and 33% with placebo.[49] In a randomized, double-blind trial in patients who had previously failed treatment with a TNF inhibitor, ACR20 response rates at 3 months were 50% with tofacitinib versus 24% with placebo.[50]

Adverse Effects – Diarrhea, nasopharyngitis, upper respiratory tract infections, headache, and hypertension are common adverse effects of tofacitinib. Aminotransferase elevations, dyslipidemia, and cytopenias have been reported; periodic monitoring is recommended. Infections, especially herpes zoster and TB, can occur. Eleven solid cancers and 1 lymphoma were diagnosed among 3328 patients who took tofacitinib with or without a DMARD for ≤12 months, compared to no solid cancers or lymphoma in 809 patients who took a placebo with or without a DMARD for 3-6 months; the significance of this finding is unclear. The tofacitinib package insert contains a boxed warning describing an increased risk of thrombosis and death with a dosage of 10 mg twice daily and emphasizes that this dosage or *Xeljanz XR* 22 mg once daily is not recommended for treatment of rheumatoid arthritis or psoriatic arthritis.[51]

Drug Interactions – Tofacitinib should not be coadministered with biologic agents or potent immunosuppressive drugs such as cyclosporine. Patients taking tofacitinib should not receive live vaccines. Tofacitinib is metabolized by CYP3A4. Strong inhibitors of CYP3A4,[12] such as ketoconazole, can increase serum concentrations of tofacitinib; its dosage should be reduced if a strong CYP3A4 inhibitor is taken concurrently. Drugs that are both moderate CYP3A4 and strong CYP2C19 inhibitors, such as fluconazole, also increase serum concentrations of tofacitinib; concurrent use requires a reduction in tofacitinib dosage. Use with strong inducers of CYP3A4, such as rifampin, can decrease tofacitinib levels and should be avoided.

Pregnancy and Lactation – There are no adequate data on the use of tofacitinib in pregnant women. In animal studies, fetocidal and teratogenic effects occurred when pregnant rats and rabbits were given tofacitinib at high doses. Tofacitinib is present in the milk of lactating rats. There are no data on the presence of tofacitinib in human breast milk or its effects on the breastfed infant or milk production. Breastfeeding is not recommended during treatment and for at least 18 hours after the last *Xeljanz* dose or 36 hours after the last *Xeljanz XR* dose.

UPADACITINIB — Upadacitinib *(Rinvoq)*, a JAK-1 selective inhibitor, was recently FDA-approved for treatment of rheumatoid arthritis.[52] In an unpublished, randomized, double-blind, placebo-controlled trial (reported only as a company press release) in 641 adults with active psoriatic arthritis who had failed to respond to ≥1 biologic DMARDs, significantly more patients achieved an ACR20 response after 12 weeks with upadacitinib than with placebo (57% with upadacitinib 15 mg and 64% with 30 mg vs 24% with placebo).

1. F Alinaghi et al. Prevalence of psoriatic arthritis in patients with psoriasis: a systematic review and meta-analysis of observational and clinical studies. J Am Acad Dermatol 2019; 80:251.
2. JA Singh et al. Special article: 2018 American College of Rheumatology/National Psoriasis Foundation guideline for the treatment of psoriatic arthritis. Arthritis Rheumatol 2019; 71:5.
3. Celecoxib safety revisited. Med Lett Drugs Ther 2016; 58:159.
4. L Gossec et al. European League Against Rheumatism (EULAR) recommendations for the management of psoriatic arthritis with pharmacological therapies: 2015 update. Ann Rheum Dis 2016; 75:499.
5. PJ Mease et al. Etanercept and methotrexate as monotherapy or in combination for psoriatic arthritis: primary results from a randomized, controlled phase III trial. Arthritis Rheumatol 2019; 71:1112.
6. C Bazzani et al. Antirheumatic drugs and reproduction in women and men with chronic arthritis. RMD Open 2015; 1: e000048.
7. JP Kaltwasser et al. Efficacy and safety of leflunomide in the treatment of psoriatic arthritis and psoriasis: a multinational, double-blind, randomized, placebo-controlled clinical trial. Arthritis Rheum 2004; 50:1939.
8. A Gottlieb et al. Guidelines of care for the management of psoriasis and psoriatic arthritis: section 2. psoriatic arthritis: overview and guidelines of care for treatment with an emphasis on the biologics. J Am Acad Dermatol 2008; 58:851.
9. D Alessa et al. Safety and efficacy of cyclosporine in psoriatic arthritis. J Psoriasis Psoriatic Arthritis 2014; 20:74.
10. AD Fraser et al. A randomised, double-blind, placebo controlled, multicentre trial of combination therapy with methotrexate plus ciclosporin in patients with active psoriatic arthritis. Ann Rheum Dis 2005; 64:859.
11. PJ Mease and AW Armstrong. Managing patients with psoriatic disease: the diagnosis and pharmacologic treatment of psoriatic arthritis in patients with psoriasis. Drugs 2014; 74:423.
12. Inhibitors and inducers of CYP enzymes and P-glycoprotein. Med Lett Drugs Ther 2019 November 6 (epub). Available at: www. medicalletter.org/downloads/CYP_PGP_Tables.pdf.
13. MB Hoffman et al. Psoriasis during pregnancy: characteristics and important management recommendations. Expert Rev Clin Immunol 2015; 11:709.
14. Apremilast (Otezla) for psoriatic arthritis. Med Lett Drugs Ther 2014; 56:41.
15. A Kavanaugh et al. Treatment of psoriatic arthritis in a phase 3 randomised, placebo-controlled trial with apremilast, an oral phosphodiesterase 4 inhibitor. Ann Rheum Dis 2014; 73:1020.
16. M Cutolo et al. A phase III, randomized, controlled trial of apremilast in patients with psoriatic arthritis: results of the PALACE 2 trial. J Rheumatol 2016; 43:1724.
17. CJ Edwards et al. Apremilast, an oral phosphodiesterase 4 inhibitor, in patients with psoriatic arthritis and current skin involvement: a phase III, randomised, controlled trial (PALACE 3). Ann Rheum Dis 2016; 75:1065.
18. A Kavanaugh et al. Long-term experience with apremilast in patients with psoriatic arthritis: 5-year results from a PALACE 1-3 pooled analysis. Arthritis Res Ther 2019; 21:118.

19. AF Wells et al. Apremilast monotherapy in DMARD-naive psoriatic arthritis patients: results of the randomized, placebo-controlled PALACE 4 trial. Rheumatology (Oxford) 2018; 57:1253.

20. P Nash et al. Early and sustained efficacy with apremilast monotherapy in biological-naive patients with psoriatic arthritis: a phase IIIB, randomised controlled trial (ACTIVE). Ann Rheum Dis 2018; 77:690.

21. R Goulabchand et al. Effect of tumour necrosis factor blockers on radiographic progression of psoriatic arthritis: a systematic review and meta-analysis of randomised controlled trials. Ann Rheum Dis 2014; 73:414.

22. D Simon et al. Effect of disease-modifying anti-rheumatic drugs on bone structure and strength in psoriatic arthritis patients. Arthritis Res Ther 2019; 21:162.

23. L Eder et al. Tumour necrosis factor α blockers are more effective than methotrexate in the inhibition of radiographic joint damage progression among patients with psoriatic arthritis. Ann Rheum Dis 2014; 73:1007.

24. AS Soubrier et al. Treatment response, drug survival and safety of anti-tumour necrosis factor α therapy in 193 patients with psoriatic arthritis: a twelve-year "real life" experience. Joint Bone Spine 2015; 82:31.

25. Certolizumab pegol (Cimzia) and ustekinumab (Stelara) for psoriatic arthritis. Med Lett Drugs Ther 2014; 56:10.

26. PJ Mease et al. Effect of certolizumab pegol on signs and symptoms in patients with psoriatic arthritis: 24-week results of a phase 3 double-blind randomised placebo-controlled study (RAPID-PsA). Ann Rheum Dis 2014; 73:48.

27. A Kavanaugh et al. Golimumab, a new human tumor necrosis factor alpha antibody, administered every four weeks as a subcutaneous injection in psoriatic arthritis: twenty-four-week efficacy and safety results of a randomized, placebo-controlled study. Arthritis Rheum 2009; 60:976.

28. F Behrens et al. Tumor necrosis factor inhibitor monotherapy vs combination with MTX in the treatment of PsA: a systematic review of the literature. Rheumatology (Oxford) 2015; 54:915.

29. LJJ van Mens et al. Achieving remission in psoriatic arthritis by early initiation of TNF inhibition: a double-blind, randomised, placebo-controlled trial of golimumab plus methotrexate versus placebo plus methotrexate. Ann Rheum Dis 2019; 78:610.

30. HMY de Jong et al. Sustained remission with methotrexate monotherapy after 22-week induction treatment with TNF-alpha inhibitor and methotrexate in early psoriatic arthritis: an open-label extension of a randomized placebo-controlled trial. Arthritis Res Ther 2019; 21:208.

31. EG Favalli et al. Eight-year retention rate of first-line tumor necrosis factor inhibitors in spondyloarthritis: a multicenter retrospective analysis. Arthritis Care Res (Hoboken) 2017; 69:867.

32. KM Fagerli et al. The role of methotrexate co-medication in TNF-inhibitor treatment in patients with psoriatic arthritis: results from 440 patients included in the NOR-DMARD study. Ann Rheum Dis 2014; 73:132.

33. PJ Mease et al. Comparative effectiveness of biologic monotherapy versus combination therapy for patients with psoriatic arthritis: results from the Corrona registry. RMD Open 2015; 1:e000181.

34. RE Kalb et al. Risk of serious infection with biologic and systemic treatment of psoriasis: results from the psoriasis longitudinal assessment and registry (PSOLAR). JAMA Dermatol 2015; 151:961.

35. AL Semble et al. Safety and tolerability of tumor necrosis factor-α inhibitors in psoriasis: a narrative review. Am J Clin Dermatol 2014; 15:37.

36. V Strand et al. Immunogenicity of biologics in chronic inflammatory diseases: a systematic review. BioDrugs 2017; 31:299.

37. IB McInnes et al. Efficacy and safety of ustekinumab in patients with active psoriatic arthritis: 1 year results of the phase 3, multicentre, double-blind, placebo-controlled PSUMMIT 1 trial. Lancet 2013; 382:780.

38. A Kavanaugh et al. Ustekinumab, an anti-IL-12/23 p40 monoclonal antibody, inhibits radiographic progression in patients with active psoriatic arthritis: results of an integrated analysis of radiographic data from the phase 3, multicentre, randomised, double-blind, placebo-controlled PSUMMIT-1 and PSUMMIT-2 trials. Ann Rheum Dis 2014; 73:1000.

39. IB McInnes et al. Secukinumab, a human anti-interleukin-17A monoclonal antibody, in patients with psoriatic arthritis (FUTURE-2); a randomised, double-blind, placebo-controlled, phase 3 trial. Lancet 2015; 386:1137.

40. PJ Mease et al. Secukinumab inhibition of interleukin-17A in patients with psoriatic arthritis. N Engl J Med 2015; 373:1329.

41. P Mease et al. Secukinumab improves active psoriatic arthritis symptoms and inhibits radiographic progression: primary results from the randomised, double-blind, phase III FUTURE 5 study. Ann Rheum Dis 2018; 77:890.

42. PJ Mease et al. Ixekizumab, an interleukin-17A specific monoclonal antibody, for the treatment of biologic-naive patients with active psoriatic arthritis: results from the 24-week randomised, double-blind, placebo-controlled and active (adalimumab)-controlled period of the phase III trial SPIRIT-P1. Ann Rheum Dis 2017; 76:79.

43. P Nash et al. Ixekizumab for the treatment of patients with active psoriatic arthritis and an inadequate response to tumour necrosis factor inhibitors: results from the 24-week randomised, double-blind, placebo-controlled period of the SPIRIT-P2 phase 3 trial. Lancet 2017; 389:2317.

44. PJ Mease et al. A head-to-head comparison of the efficacy and safety of ixekizumab and adalimumab in biological-naive patients with active psoriatic arthritis: 24-week results of a randomised, open-label, blinded-assessor trial. Ann Rheum Dis 2019 Sept 28 (epub).

45. P Mease et al. Abatacept in the treatment of patients with psoriatic arthritis: results of a six-month, multicenter, randomized, double-blind, placebo-controlled, phase II trial. Arthritis Rheum 2011; 63:939.

46. PJ Mease et al. Efficacy and safety of abatacept, a T-cell modulator, in a randomised, double-blind, placebo-controlled, phase III study in psoriatic arthritis. Ann Rheum Dis 2017; 76:1550.

47. DC Butler et al. Safety of dermatologic medications in pregnancy and lactation: part II: lactation. J Am Acad Dermatol 2014; 70:417.

48. Tofacitinib (Xeljanz) for rheumatoid arthritis. Med Lett Drugs Ther 2013; 55:1.

49. P Mease et al. Tofacitinib or adalimumab versus placebo for psoriatic arthritis. N Engl J Med 2017; 377:1537.

50. D Gladman et al. Tofacitinib for psoriatic arthritis in patients with an inadequate response to TNF inhibitors. N Engl J Med 2017; 377:1525.
51. In brief: risk of pulmonary thromboembolism and death with tofacitinib (Xeljanz). Med Lett Drugs Ther 2019; 61:136.
52. Upadacitinib (Rinvoq) – A new JAK inhibitor for rheumatoid arthritis. Med Lett Drugs Ther 2019; 61:183.

OTC DRUGS FOR
Seasonal Allergies

Original publication date – April 2019

Patients with seasonal allergies often experience nasal itching and congestion, sneezing, rhinorrhea, and itchy, watery eyes. Oral, intranasal, and ophthalmic preparations are widely available over the counter (OTC) for relief of symptoms. Prescription products for management of allergic rhinitis and allergic conjunctivitis are reviewed separately.[1]

INTRANASAL CORTICOSTEROIDS — Intranasal corticosteroids are the most effective drugs available for prevention and treatment of allergic rhinitis symptoms. They are modestly effective in reducing ocular symptoms (itching, tearing, redness).[2] All OTC intranasal corticosteroids appear to be similar in efficacy. Their onset of action typically occurs within 12 hours, but maximal effects may not be achieved for ≥7 days.

Adverse Effects — Intranasal corticosteroids can cause dryness, irritation, burning, and bleeding of the nasal mucosa, sore throat, and headache. Ulceration, mucosal atrophy, septal perforation, intranasal and/or oropharyngeal infection, and increased intraocular pressure have been reported. Use of some intranasal corticosteroids for ≥12 months in children has been associated with small decreases in growth velocity.[3,4]

ANTIHISTAMINES — **Oral first-generation** H_1-antihistamines such as diphenhydramine (*Benadryl*, and generics) can cause sedation and

---

Recommendations for OTC Treatment of Seasonal Allergies

- ► Intranasal corticosteroids are the most effective drugs available for prevention and treatment of allergic rhinitis symptoms; they are modestly effective in reducing ocular symptoms.
- ► Oral first-generation H_1-antihistamines are not recommended because they can cause CNS impairment and sedation.
- ► Oral second-generation H_1-antihistamines are the preferred first-line treatment for mild episodic allergic rhinitis symptoms.
- ► Oral and intranasal decongestants only relieve congestion; an oral decongestant is often used with an oral H_1-antihistamine for treatment of allergic rhinitis symptoms.
- ► Intranasal and ophthalmic decongestants can cause rebound nasal congestion and hyperemia with prolonged use (>3-5 days).
- ► Ophthalmic antihistamines are at least as effective as oral second-generation H_1-antihistamines for treatment of allergic conjunctivitis and are recommended for patients who have primarily ocular symptoms.

CNS impairment and are generally not recommended for treatment of allergic rhinitis.[5]

Oral second-generation H_1-antihistamines are preferred for first-line treatment of mild episodic allergic rhinitis symptoms. They are effective for treatment of nasal itching, sneezing, and rhinorrhea; they are less effective for nasal congestion. They can also reduce ocular symptoms.

Addition of an oral second-generation H_1-antihistamine to an intranasal corticosteroid is not more effective than an intranasal corticosteroid alone.

Intranasal H_1-antihistamines have a rapid onset of action and their clinical efficacy in allergic rhinitis, including relief of nasal congestion, is equal or superior to that of oral H_1-antihistamines, but they are only available with a prescription.

Adverse Effects — Oral first-generation H_1-antihistamines can interfere with learning and memory, impair performance, decrease work productivity, and increase the risk of motor vehicle accidents and on-the-job injuries. When these drugs are taken at night, adverse effects on wakefulness and psychomotor performance can persist into the next day.[6] Cumulative exposure to first-generation H_1-antihistamines with strong anticholinergic properties has been associated with dementia.[7]

Oral second-generation H_1-antihistamines penetrate poorly into the CNS and are significantly less likely than first-generation drugs to cause CNS impairment and sedation.[8,9] Fexofenadine does not cause sedation or CNS impairment, even at higher-than-recommended doses. Loratadine and desloratadine (*Clarinex*, and others; only available with a prescription) do not cause CNS impairment or sedation at recommended doses, but they may cause sedation at higher doses. Cetirizine and levocetirizine can cause sedation at recommended doses.[1]

Intranasal H_1-antihistamines can cause dysgeusia, nasal discomfort, epistaxis, headache, and sedation.

DECONGESTANTS — The **oral** decongestant pseudoephedrine (*Sudafed*, and others) and **intranasal** decongestants such as oxymetazoline (*Afrin*, and generics) act as vasoconstrictors in the nasal mucosa, primarily through stimulation of alpha-1 adrenergic receptors on venous sinusoids. They only relieve nasal congestion, not sneezing, nasal itching, or rhinorrhea, and tolerance to their decongestant effects can occur. Phenylephrine (*Sudafed PE*, and others) has replaced pseudoephedrine in many OTC products because illicit pseudoephedrine use has resulted in sales restrictions, but phenylephrine is not effective for treatment of nasal congestion.[10,11] An oral decongestant is often used in combination with an oral H_1-antihistamine for treatment of allergic rhinitis symptoms.

Adverse Effects — **Oral** decongestants can cause insomnia, excitability, headache, nervousness, anorexia, palpitations, tachycardia, arrhythmias, hypertension, nausea, vomiting, and urinary retention. These drugs should be used cautiously in patients with cardiovascular disease,

OTC Drugs for Seasonal Allergies

Table 1. Some OTC Nasal Sprays for Allergic Rhinitis

Drug	Some Formulations
Corticosteroids	
Budesonide[2] – *Rhinocort Allergy* (Johnson & Johnson) *Children's Rhinocort Allergy*	Metered-dose pump spray (32 mcg/spray) 60, 120 sprays (5, 8.43 mL bottles)[3]
Fluticasone furoate – *Flonase Sensimist Allergy Relief* (GSK)[6] *Children's Flonase Sensimist Allergy Relief*[6]	Metered-dose pump spray (27.5 mcg/spray) 60, 120 sprays (5.9, 15.8 mL bottles)[3]
Fluticasone propionate[2] – *Flonase Allergy Relief* (GSK)[6,7] *Children's Flonase Allergy Relief*[6,7]	Metered-dose pump spray (50 mcg/spray) 60, 120 sprays (9.9, 15.8 mL bottles)[3]
Triamcinolone acetonide[2] – *Nasacort Allergy 24HR* (Sanofi)[6] *Children's Nasacort Allergy 24HR*[6]	Metered-dose pump spray (55 mcg/spray) 60, 120 sprays (10.8, 16.9 mL bottles)[3]
Mast Cell Stabilizer	
Cromolyn sodium[2] – *Nasalcrom* (Prestige)[6]	Metered-dose pump spray (5.2 mg/spray) 100, 200 sprays (13, 26 mL bottles)

1. Cost according to target.com or walgreens.com. Accessed April 11, 2019.
2. Individual retailers may have their own OTC generic products.
3. Children's product is only available in the smaller size bottle.
4. A dose of 2 sprays should only be used until symptoms improve, then the dose should be reduced to 1 spray/nostril.

hypertension, diabetes, hyperthyroidism, closed-angle glaucoma, or bladder neck obstruction.

Intranasal decongestants are less likely than oral decongestants to cause systemic adverse effects, but they can cause stinging, burning, and dryness of the nose and throat. To avoid rebound nasal congestion, they should not be used as monotherapy for >3-5 consecutive days.

MAST CELL STABILIZER — Use of intranasal cromolyn sodium before allergen exposure inhibits mast cell degranulation and mediator release, preventing allergic rhinitis symptoms. It should be started 1-2

Usual Dosage	Cost[1]
6-11 yrs: 1-2 sprays per nostril once/day[4,5] ≥12 yrs: 2 sprays per nostril once/day[4,5]	$13.99/5 mL 12.99/5 mL
2-11 yrs: 1 spray per nostril once/day[5] ≥12 yrs: 2 sprays per nostril once/day x 7 days, then 1-2 sprays per nostril once/day[4,5]	13.99/5.9 mL 15.99/5.9 mL
4-11 yrs: 1 spray per nostril once/day[5] ≥12 yrs: 2 sprays per nostril once/day x 7 days, then 1-2 sprays per nostril once/day[4,5]	13.99/9.9 mL 13.99/9.9 mL
2-5 yrs: 1 spray per nostril once/day[5] 6-11 yrs: 1-2 sprays per nostril once/day[4,5] ≥12 yrs: 2 sprays per nostril once/day[4,5]	12.99/10.8 mL 12.99/10.8 mL
≥2 yrs: 1 spray per nostril tid-qid	9.99/13 mL

5. OTC intranasal corticosteroids should not be used daily for >2 months/year in patients <12 years old or for >6 months in those ≥12 years old without consulting a physician.
6. Contains benzalkonium chloride (preservative), which can cause irritation of the nasal mucosa.
7. Contains alcohol, which may cause dryness.

weeks before exposure to the allergen and must be used 3-4 times daily. Intranasal cromolyn sodium is less effective than oral second-generation H_1-antihistamines and intranasal corticosteroids.[12] Nasal stinging can occur.

NASAL SALINE – Nasal saline sprays and drops can be used to relieve nasal dryness and congestion. Nasal irrigations administered by neti pot, squeeze bottle, or bulb syringe can help expel mucus and relieve congestion. Premade saline solutions and kits are available OTC. Patients should be cautioned to use sterile, distilled, or previously boiled water to prepare solutions for nasal irrigation. Use of tap water has been associated with primary amebic meningoencephalitis.

Table 2. Some OTC Oral Second-Generation H₁-Antihistamines and Combinations for Allergic Rhinitis[1]

Drug	Some Formulations
H₁-Antihistamines	
Cetirizine[3,4] –	
Zyrtec Allergy (Johnson & Johnson)	10 mg tabs, caps, disintegrating tabs
Children's Zyrtec Allergy	10 mg disintegrating tabs; 5 mg/5 mL syrup
Fexofenadine[3,4] –	
Allegra Allergy 24HR (Sanofi)	180 mg tabs, caps
Children's Allegra Allergy 12HR	30 mg disintegrating tabs; 30 mg/5 mL susp
Levocetirizine[3,4] –	
Xyzal Allergy 24HR (Sanofi)	5 mg tabs
Children's Xyzal Allergy 24HR	2.5 mg/5 mL soln
Loratadine[3] –	
Alavert (Pfizer)	10 mg disintegrating tabs
Claritin 12 Hour (Bayer)	5 mg disintegrating tabs
Claritin 24 Hour	10 mg tabs, caps, disintegrating tabs
Children's Claritin 12 Hour	5 mg chewable tabs
Children's Claritin 24 Hour	5 mg chewable tabs, disintegrating tabs; 10 mg disintegrating tabs; 1 mg/mL syrup
H₁-Antihistamine/Decongestant Combinations	
Cetirizine/pseudoephedrine[3,5] – Zyrtec-D (Johnson & Johnson)	5 mg/120 mg ER tabs
Fexofenadine/pseudoephedrine[3,5] – Allegra-D 24HR (Sanofi)	180 mg/240 mg ER tabs
Loratadine/pseudoephedrine[3,5] –	
Alavert D-12 Hour (Pfizer)	5 mg/120 mg ER tabs
Claritin-D 12 Hour (Bayer)	
Claritin-D 24 Hour	10 mg/240 mg ER tabs

ER = extended-release
1. Dosage adjustments may be needed for renal or hepatic impairment.
2. Cost according to cvs.com or walmart.com. Accessed April 11, 2019.

Usual Dosage	Cost[2]
2-5 yrs: 2.5 or 5 mg once/day or 2.5 mg bid 6-11 yrs: 5 or 10 mg once/day 12-64 yrs: 10 mg once/day ≥65 yrs: 5 mg once/day	$18.99/30 tabs 15.49/4 oz
2-11 yrs: 30 mg bid 12-64 yrs: 180 mg once/day	18.99/30 tabs 10.79/4 oz
2-5 yrs: 1.25 mg once/day 6-11 yrs: 2.5 mg once/day 12-64 yrs: 5 mg once/day	26.44/80 tabs 10.99/5 oz
2-5 yrs: 5 mg once/day ≥6 yrs: 5 mg bid or 10 mg once/day	18.89/60 tabs 19.99/30 tabs 19.99/30 tabs 8.59/10 tabs 9.82/4 oz
12-64 yrs: 1 tab bid	20.96/24 tabs
12-64 yrs: 1 tab once/day	12.89/15 tabs
≥12 yrs: 1 tab bid ≥12 yrs: 1 tab once/day	14.97/24 tabs 18.88/30 tabs 12.49/10 tabs

3. Individual retailers may have their own OTC generic products.
4. The prescription product is approved for use in children ≥6 months old.
5. Products containing pseudoephedrine are subject to sales restrictions because of illicit use.

Table 3. Some OTC Ophthalmic Drugs for Allergic Conjunctivitis	
Drug	**Some Formulations**
Decongestants	
Naphazoline – *Clear Eyes Redness Relief* (Prestige)	0.012%[3] (10 mL)
Tetrahydrozoline[4] – *Visine A.C.*[5] (Johnson & Johnson)	0.05%[3] (15, 30 mL)
H₁-Antihistamine	
Ketotifen[4] – *Alaway* (Bausch + Lomb)	0.025%[3] (10 mL)
Zaditor (Alcon)	0.025%[3] (5 mL)
H₁-Antihistamine/Decongestant Combination	
Pheniramine/naphazoline – *Naphcon-A* (Alcon)	0.3%/0.025%[3] (15 mL)
Opcon-A (Bausch + Lomb)	0.3%/0.027%[3] (15 mL)
Visine-A (Johnson & Johnson)	0.3%/0.025%[3] (15 mL)

1. Patients who experience stinging or burning should try refrigerating the drug before use.
2. Cost according to target.com. Accessed April 11, 2019.
3. Contains benzalkonium chloride (preservative), which may cause irritation in some patients.

PREGNANCY — In a meta-analysis that included >50,000 women, exposure to **H₁-antihistamines** during the first trimester of pregnancy was not associated with an increased risk of major malformations, spontaneous abortions, prematurity, or low birth weight.[13] The oral second-generation H₁-antihistamines **loratidine** and **cetirizine** are preferred for use in pregnant women. **Nasal saline**, **cromolyn sodium**, and **intranasal corticosteroids** are generally considered safe for treatment of allergic rhinitis in pregnant women.[14]

Oral decongestants are generally not recommended for treatment of allergic rhinitis in pregnant women; oral pseudoephedrine should not be used during the first trimester. An **intranasal decongestant** can be used for short-term treatment (3-5 days) of congestion in pregnant women.

ALLERGIC CONJUNCTIVITIS — Allergic conjunctivitis symptoms such as itching, redness, tearing, and photophobia occur in most patients with seasonal allergies. Nonpharmacologic management includes allergen

Usual Dosage[1]	Cost[2]
1-2 drops up to qid	$3.29/10 mL
≥6 yrs: 1-2 drops up to qid	3.84/15 mL
>3 yrs: 1 drop bid (q8-12h)	10.99/10 mL
	12.99/5 mL
≥6 yrs: 1-2 drops up to qid	10.59/15 mL
	5.49/15 mL
	5.99/15 mL

4. Individual retailers may have their own generic products.
5. Also contains zinc sulfate 0.25%, which is an astringent.

identification and avoidance, use of cool compresses, and avoidance of eye rubbing and contact lens wearing during symptomatic periods.

Ophthalmic H$_1$-antihistamines are at least as effective as oral second-generation H$_1$-antihistamines for treatment of allergic conjunctivitis, and they have a faster onset of action (within a few minutes). They can be used as monotherapy in patients who have primarily ocular symptoms.[15,16] Ketotifen *(Alaway, Zaditor)*, which is marketed as having both H$_1$-antihistamine and mast-cell-stabilizing activity, is the only ophthalmic antihistamine available OTC. Other dual-acting ophthalmic H$_1$-antihistamine and mast-cell-stabilizing drugs, such as olopatadine *(Patanol, Pataday, Pazeo)* and azelastine, are only available with a prescription.

Ophthalmic decongestants such as naphazoline reduce erythema, congestion, itching, and eyelid edema, but they have a short duration of action and can cause burning and stinging. They should only be used short-term to avoid rebound hyperemia. The OTC ophthalmic **H₁-antihistamine/decongestant combination** pheniramine/naphazoline has similar adverse effects.

The **ophthalmic mast cell stabilizer** cromolyn sodium has a slower onset of action than ophthalmic H₁-antihistamines and is mostly used for treatment of mild to moderate ocular symptoms. It is FDA-approved for treatment of vernal keratoconjunctivitis, conjunctivitis, and keratitis and is only available with a prescription.

Ophthalmic corticosteroids such as loteprednol (*Lotemax*, and others) and prednisone, which are only available with a prescription, can be considered for use in allergic conjunctivitis that fails to respond to other medications.

1. Drugs for allergic disorders. Med Lett Drugs Ther 2017; 59:71.
2. OTC fluticasone furoate nasal spray (Flonase Sensimist) for allergic rhinitis. Med Lett Drugs Ther 2017; 59:e70.
3. L Lasmar et al. Growth velocity in prepubertal children using both inhaled and intranasal corticosteroids. Ann Allergy Asthma Immunol 2016; 116:368.
4. DJ Mener et al. Topical intranasal corticosteroids and growth velocity in children: a meta-analysis. Int Forum Allergy Rhinol 2015; 5:95.
5. MS Dykewicz et al. Treatment of seasonal allergic rhinitis: an evidence-based focused 2017 guideline update. Ann Allergy Asthma Immunol 2017; 119:489.
6. Y Katayose et al. Carryover effect on next-day sleepiness and psychomotor performance of nighttime administered antihistaminic drugs: a randomized controlled trial. Hum Psychopharmacol 2012; 27:428.
7. K Richardson et al. Anticholinergic drugs and risk of dementia: case-control study. BMJ 2018; 361:k1315.
8. FE Simons and KJ Simons. Histamine and H1-antihistamines: celebrating a century of progress. J Allergy Clin Immunol 2011; 128:1139.
9. MK Church et al. Risk of first-generation H(1)-antihistamines: a GA(2)LEN position paper. Allergy 2010; 65:459.
10. In brief: oral phenylephrine for nasal congestion. Med Lett Drugs Ther 2015; 57:174.
11. EO Meltzer et al. Oral phenylephrine HCl for nasal congestion in seasonal allergic rhinitis: a randomized, open-label, placebo-controlled study. J Allergy Clin Immunol Pract 2015; 3:702.

12. B Lange et al. Efficacy, cost-effectiveness, and tolerability of mometasone furoate, levo-cabastine, and disodium cromoglycate nasal sprays in the treatment of seasonal allergic rhinitis. Ann Allergy Asthma Immunol 2005; 95:272.
13. F Etwel et al. The risk of adverse pregnancy outcome after first trimester exposure to H1-antihistamines: a systematic review and meta-analysis. Drug Saf 2017; 40:121.
14. I Pali-Schöll et al. Allergic diseases and asthma in pregnancy, a secondary publication. World Allergy Organ J 2017; 10:10.
15. DM Varu et al. Conjuctivitis preferred practice pattern. Ophthalmology 2019; 126:p94.
16. M Shaker and E Salcone. An update on ocular allergy. Curr Opin Allergy Clin Immunol 2016; 16:505.

DRUGS FOR
Smoking Cessation

Original publication date – July 2019

Smoking tobacco remains the primary preventable cause of death in the US. Smoking cessation often requires both pharmacotherapy and behavioral support.[1,2]

NICOTINE REPLACEMENT — All FDA-approved nicotine replacement therapies (NRTs) deliver nicotine to nicotinic acetylcholine receptors in the central nervous system (CNS) in a lower dose and at a substantially slower rate than tobacco cigarettes and electronic nicotine delivery systems. Nicotine undergoes extensive first-pass metabolism, which limits its effectiveness in oral formulations. Nicotine gum, lozenges, and patches are available over the counter in the US for persons ≥18 years old; they appear to be as effective as nicotine products that require a prescription (oral inhaler and nasal spray).

Transdermal – Nicotine **patches** deliver nicotine continuously, but they require 6-8 hours to achieve peak serum concentrations and deliver nicotine to the CNS more slowly than any other NRT.

Rapid Onset – Nicotine from a **gum, lozenge, or oral inhaler** is absorbed through the buccal mucosa. Serum concentrations peak in 20-60 minutes. If nicotine is swallowed, first-pass metabolism reduces its bioavailability.

Summary: Drugs for Smoking Cessation

▶ Smoking cessation can be safely and effectively achieved with pharmaco-therapy and behavioral support.
▶ All nicotine replacement therapies (NRTs) appear to be about equally effective; combining a patch and a rapid-onset formulation is more effective than either one alone.
▶ Bupropion SR is as effective as single NRT.
▶ Varenicline is the most effective monotherapy and is as effective as combination NRT.
▶ The optimal duration of treatment is not clear; most patients should receive at least 3-6 months of effective therapy.
▶ The efficacy and safety of using electronic cigarettes for smoking cessation have not been established.

Nicotine **nasal spray** is the fastest-acting of all NRTs (but still much slower than cigarettes); serum concentrations peak in 4-15 minutes. Patients report that relief of nicotine withdrawal symptoms is faster with the nasal spray than with other NRT formulations.

When used as monotherapy, rapid-onset NRT should be taken on a regular schedule to prevent nicotine withdrawal symptoms.

Efficacy – All NRTs increase smoking cessation rates by 50-60%. In the short term, they may also decrease weight gain associated with smoking cessation.[3,4] The combination of a patch and a rapid-onset formulation is more effective than either one alone.[5]

Adverse Effects – The nicotine **transdermal patch** is generally well tolerated, but pruritus at the application site, insomnia, and vivid dreams can occur. Removing the patch at bedtime can minimize or eliminate vivid dreams and other sleep disturbances. Nicotine **gum** can cause flat-ulence, indigestion, nausea, unpleasant taste, hiccups, and a sore mouth, throat, and jaw. Nicotine **lozenges** can cause mouth irritation, heartburn, hiccups, and nausea. The nicotine **oral inhaler** can cause mild mouth and throat irritation and cough; tolerance to the irritating effects usually develops within one or two days. Nicotine **nasal spray** can cause transient burning and stinging of the nasal mucosa, throat irritation, flushing, coughing, sneezing, lacrimation, rhinorrhea, and nausea; these adverse effects are a common cause of discontinuation.

Drug Interactions – Nicotine does not induce or inhibit CYP450 enzymes to a clinically significant extent. Tobacco smoke, not nicotine itself, induces CYP1A2, CYP2E1, and some uridine diphosphate-glucuronosyltransferases (UGTs); it may increase the metabolism and decrease the efficacy of drugs that are substrates of these enzymes, such as clozapine (*Clozaril,* and others), olanzapine (*Zyprexa,* and generics), and propranolol (*Inderal,* and others).[6-8] The dosages of these drugs may need to be reduced when patients stop smoking.

BUPROPION — Bupropion, which is used mainly for treatment of depression, has some nicotinic-receptor-blocking activity and may also aid smoking cessation by inhibiting dopamine reuptake. A sustained-release (SR) formulation of bupropion *(Zyban)* is FDA-approved as a smoking cessation aid. Bupropion SR should be started 7-14 days before the target quit date to allow serum concentrations to reach steady state.

Efficacy – Bupropion SR has doubled smoking cessation rates compared to placebo in short-term trials. It has been as effective as single NRT in increasing long-term (≥6 months) smoking cessation rates and decreasing weight gain.[9]

Adverse Effects – Bupropion is generally well tolerated. The most common adverse effects in clinical trials were insomnia and dry mouth. Headache, nausea, and anxiety can also occur.[10] Bupropion SR has been associated with a dose-related increase in the risk of seizures; patients with a history of seizure, stroke, brain tumor, severe head injury, anorexia nervosa, or bulimia should not take bupropion.

Drug Interactions – Bupropion is primarily metabolized by CYP2B6 to hydroxybupropion, its most active metabolite. Drugs that are inhibitors or

Drugs for Smoking Cessation

Drug	Some Formulations
Table 1. Some Drugs for Smoking Cessation	
Nicotine Replacement Therapies (NRTs)	
Nicotine transdermal patch[4] – generic *NicoDerm CQ* (GSK)	7, 14, 21 mg/24 hr patches
Nicotine polacrilex gum[4] – generic *Nicorette* Gum (GSK)	2, 4 mg/pieces
Nicotine polacrilex lozenge[4,9] – generic *Nicorette* Lozenge (GSK)	2, 4 mg/lozenges
Nicotine oral inhaler – *Nicotrol* (Pfizer)	10 mg cartridges
Nicotine nasal spray – *Nicotrol NS* (Pfizer)	200 sprays/10 mL bottles (0.5 mg/spray)
Dopaminergic-Noradrenergic Reuptake Inhibitor	
Bupropion SR – generic *Wellbutrin SR* (GSK)[14] *Zyban* (GSK)	100, 150, 200 mg SR tabs[13] 150 mg SR tabs
Nicotinic Receptor Partial Agonist	
Varenicline tartrate – *Chantix* (Pfizer)	0.5, 1 mg tabs

SR = sustained-release
1. Dosage reductions may be needed for hepatic or renal impairment.
2. Patients should receive a minimum of 3-6 months of effective therapy. In general, the dosage of NRTs can be tapered at the end of treatment; bupropion SR and varenicline can usually be stopped without a gradual dosage reduction, but some clinicians recommend a taper.
3. Approximate WAC for 30 days' treatment at the lowest usual dosage. WAC = wholesaler acquisition cost, or manufacturer's published price to wholesalers; WAC represents a published catalogue or list price and may not represent an actual transactional price. Source: AnalySource® Monthly. June 5, 2019. Reprinted with permission by First Databank, Inc. All rights reserved. ©2019. www.fdbhealth.com/policies/drug-pricing-policy.
4. Available over the counter (OTC) for persons ≥18 years old.
5. See expanded table for dosage titration instructions, available at: medicalletter.org/TML-article-1576c.

inducers of CYP2B6 may alter serum concentrations of hydroxybupropion, resulting in decreased efficacy or toxicity. Bupropion and hydroxybupropion inhibit CYP2D6; many antidepressants, antipsychotics, beta blockers, and class 1C antiarrhythmics are CYP2D6 substrates and should be used with caution in patients taking bupropion.[6] Use of bupropion with a monoamine oxidase (MAO) inhibitor or within 2 weeks of stopping one is contraindicated. Drugs that lower the seizure threshold, such as tricyclic antidepressants or theophylline, should be used with caution.

Usual Adult Dosage[1,2]	Cost[3]
1 patch/day[5]	$44.20[6]
	63.30[6]
8-24 pieces/day[5,7,8]	60.00
	101.30
8-20 lozenges/day[5,7,10]	89.60
	99.60
4-16 cartridges/day[5]	416.60[11]
2 sprays 8-40x/day (max 10 sprays/hr)[4]	328.00[12]
150 mg PO once/day x 3 days, then 150 mg PO bid	21.00
	445.30
	247.80
0.5 mg PO once/day x 3 days, then 0.5 mg bid on days 4-7, then 1 mg bid	451.40

6. Cost of 28 transdermal patches.
7. Eating or drinking within 15 minutes of using a gum or lozenge should be avoided.
8. A second piece of gum can be used within one hour. Continuously chewing one piece after another is not recommended.
9. Also available in a mini-lozenge.
10. Maximum of 5 lozenges in 6 hours or 20 lozenges/day. Use of more than one lozenge at a time or continuously using one after another is not recommended.
11. Cost of 168 10-mg cartridges; each cartridge delivers 4 mg of nicotine.
12. Cost of 3 10-mL bottles.
13. Only the generic 150-mg SR tablets are FDA-approved as a smoking cessation aid.
14. Not FDA-approved as a smoking cessation aid.

VARENICLINE — Varenicline tartrate *(Chantix)*, a nicotinic receptor partial agonist, is FDA-approved as a smoking cessation aid.[11] It selectively binds to $\alpha_4\beta_2$ neuronal nicotinic acetylcholine receptors, which mediate release of dopamine in the brain, relieving cravings and withdrawal symptoms during abstinence. Varenicline has greater affinity for the $\alpha_4\beta_2$ receptor than nicotine, reducing the reward of smoking. Varenicline should be started 7 days before the target quit date to allow serum concentrations to reach steady state.

Efficacy – In randomized controlled trials, including both short-term trials and some lasting for up to one year, varenicline was more effective than single NRT or bupropion and as effective as combination NRT (nicotine patch plus a rapid-onset NRT) in increasing smoking cessation rates.[12,13] In one open-label trial in 1086 smokers, smoking cessation rates were similar with varenicline, combination NRT, and a nicotine patch alone at 26 and 52 weeks; the level of nicotine dependence among smokers at enrollment in the trial was relatively low.[14]

In an unpublished study, summarized in the package insert, 312 smokers 12-19 years old were randomized to receive weight-based varenicline or placebo for 12 weeks, followed by 40 weeks of no treatment; all patients received counseling during the study. No improvement in smoking abstinence rates was observed at weeks 9-12, compared to placebo. Varenicline is not recommended for use in patients ≤16 years old.

Adverse Effects – Varenicline is generally well tolerated. The most common adverse effects in clinical trials were nausea, sleep disturbances, abnormal dreams, headache, constipation, vomiting, and flatulence. In observational studies, use of varenicline has been associated with neuropsychiatric symptoms, exacerbations of pre-existing psychiatric disorders, suicidal behavior, and an increased rate of cardiovascular events.[15] However, in a retrospective cohort study in about 165,000 patients, varenicline was not associated with an increased risk of any cardiovascular or neuropsychiatric event, compared to NRT or bupropion.[16] Recent analyses of clinical trials have found no increase in suicidal behavior in patients treated with varenicline, compared to those treated with NRT, bupropion, or placebo.[17] Varenicline has increased smoking cessation rates in patients with psychiatric disorders without causing significant neuropsychiatric adverse effects.[18,19]

Drug Interactions – Varenicline has no clinically significant drug interactions.

A COMPARATIVE CLINICAL TRIAL — In a double-blind postmarketing trial (EAGLES), 8144 motivated-to-quit smokers with or without a diagnosed psychiatric disorder were randomized to receive varenicline 1 mg twice daily, bupropion SR 150 mg twice daily, a transdermal nicotine patch 21 mg daily with taper, or placebo for 12 weeks, followed by 12 weeks of no treatment. Continuous abstinence rates were significantly higher with all active treatments than with placebo (see Table 2). Varenicline was the most effective treatment; bupropion and the nicotine patch were similar in efficacy.

Patients without a psychiatric disorder who received active treatment had fewer neuropsychiatric events than those who received placebo. In patients with a psychiatric disorder, those who received active treatment had slightly higher rates of neuropsychiatric events than those who received placebo (6.5% with varenicline, 6.7% with bupropion SR, and 5.2% with the nicotine patch, vs 4.9% with placebo). Most events were transient and had no serious consequences.[20] Based on the outcomes of the EAGLES trial, the FDA approved removal of the boxed warning about serious neuropsychiatric events from the labels of varenicline and bupropion.

COMBINATION THERAPY — Combined use of NRTs, especially a patch with a rapid-acting formulation, has generally been more effective than single NRT for smoking cessation.[5] NRT in combination with other drugs has also been beneficial.

In a randomized trial in 127 smokers with comorbid conditions, smoking abstinence rates at 26 weeks were significantly higher with a **nicotine patch combined with a nicotine oral inhaler ad libitum and bupropion SR** than with a standard 10-week tapering regimen with the patch alone (35% vs 19%).[21]

In a randomized trial in 446 smokers that included a 12-week treatment period and a 12-week follow-up, continuous abstinence rates with **varenicline plus a nicotine patch** were significantly higher than with varenicline alone at 12 weeks (55.4% vs 40.9%) and 24 weeks (49.0% vs 32.6%).[22]

Table 2. EAGLES Trial Efficacy Results[1]	
	Varenicline
All Patients	**(n=2037)**
Continuous abstinence, week 9-12	33.5%*
Continuous abstinence, week 9-24	21.8%*
Psychiatric Cohort	**(n=1032)**
Continuous abstinence, week 9-12	29.2%*
Continuous abstinence, week 9-24	18.3%*
Non-Psychiatric Cohort	**(n=1005)**
Continuous abstinence, week 9-12	38.0%*
Continuous abstinence, week 9-24	25.5%*

*statistically significant difference vs all other treatments
1. RM Anthenelli et al. Lancet 2016; 387:2507.

In a randomized trial in 506 smokers, prolonged abstinence rates were higher with **varenicline plus bupropion SR** than with varenicline alone at 12 weeks (53.0% vs 43.2%), 26 weeks (36.6% vs 27.6%), and 52 weeks (30.9% vs 24.5%), but the differences were only statistically significant at 12 and 26 weeks.[23]

In a prospective, placebo-controlled trial in 122 male smokers who had not achieved a >50% reduction in smoking with the nicotine patch (nonresponders), there was no significant difference in continuous abstinence rates at weeks 8-11 between those who received **varenicline plus bupropion SR** and those who received varenicline alone (32.1% vs 45.6%). Combination treatment was, however, significantly more effective than monotherapy in a subgroup of nonresponders who were highly nicotine dependent at baseline (66.7% vs 36.4%).[24]

DURATION OF TREATMENT — Longer-duration pharmacotherapy may improve smoking cessation rates.[25] Most patients should receive a minimum of 3-6 months of effective therapy. In one randomized trial in 525 treatment-seeking smokers, use of the nicotine patch for up to 1

Bupropion SR	Nicotine Patch	Placebo
(n=2034)	(n=2038)	(n=2035)
22.6%[†]	23.4%[†]	12.5%
16.2%[†]	15.7%[†]	9.4%
(n=1033)	(n=1025)	(n=1026)
19.3%[†]	20.4%[†]	11.4%
13.7%[†]	13.0%[†]	8.3%
(n=1001)	(n=1013)	(n=1009)
26.1%[†]	26.4%[†]	13.7%
18.8%[†]	18.5%[†]	10.5%

[†]statistically significant difference vs placebo only

year was safe, but was not more effective than 24 weeks of treatment.[26] In general, the dosage of NRTs can be tapered at the end of treatment; bupropion SR and varenicline can usually be stopped without a gradual dosage reduction, but some clinicians recommend a taper.

SMOKING CESSATION STRATEGIES – The standard practice is to advise patients that abrupt smoking cessation is more effective than gradual withdrawal, but studies comparing the 2 strategies have produced mixed results.[27]

A meta-analysis of 10 trials found that reducing cigarette consumption before the target quit date and quitting abruptly produced comparable smoking abstinence rates.[28]

In a randomized noninferiority trial in 697 adult smokers who received NRT, abrupt cessation was more likely than gradual withdrawal (75% reduction in baseline smoking over 2 weeks before a planned quit date) to result in abstinence at 4 weeks (49.0% vs 39.2%) and 6 months (22.0% vs 15.5%) after the target quit date.[29]

Other strategies that were found to have minimal to moderate success in stopping or reducing smoking include mailing free nicotine patches to willing-to-quit smokers, providing financial incentives to quit smoking, and using cigarettes with reduced nicotine content.[30-33]

ELECTRONIC NICOTINE DELIVERY SYSTEMS — Electronic cigarettes, also called e-cigarettes, are advertised as a safer, more convenient, and socially acceptable alternative to tobacco cigarettes. They are not approved by the FDA as smoking cessation aids. E-cigarettes are battery-operated devices that typically contain a heating element (atomizer) and a reservoir of liquid (usually nicotine dissolved in propylene glycol and/or glycerin). When the user inhales or activates the device with a button, the liquid nicotine is vaporized into a visible mist.

Clinical Studies – In a randomized trial in 657 tobacco cigarette smokers who wanted to quit, abstinence rates at 6 months were not significantly higher with a 16-mg nicotine e-cigarette (7.3%) than with a 21-mg nicotine patch (5.8%) or placebo e-cigarette device (4.1%).[34]

In a randomized trial in 886 smokers that compared use of the participant's choice of NRT, including combinations, with use of e-cigarettes for smoking cessation, the abstinence rate at 52 weeks was significantly higher in the e-cigarette group than in the NRT group (18.0% vs 9.9%). Among patients who reported abstinence at 52 weeks, significantly more of those in the e-cigarette group were still using their assigned product at 52 weeks (80% vs 9% in the NRT group). Patients using an e-cigarette had greater declines from baseline in cough and phlegm production at 52 weeks than those using NRT.[35]

In a meta-analysis of 38 trials in tobacco cigarette smokers, including some who wanted to quit, those who used e-cigarettes were 28% less likely to quit smoking tobacco cigarettes than those who did not use e-cigarettes.[36]

Adverse Effects – The long-term safety of e-cigarettes is unknown.[37,38] The most common adverse effects reported during clinical trials were mouth and throat irritation and dry cough. Daily e-cigarette use, adjusted for use of tobacco cigarettes, has been associated with myocardial infarction.[39] Lipoid pneumonia has been reported.[40] In nonsmokers, repeated exposure to nicotine in e-cigarettes could lead to nicotine dependence. Use of e-cigarettes by adolescents has been increasing and is particularly concerning because it could lead to subsequent use of tobacco cigarettes.[41]

Update – According to the CDC, as of November 20, 2019, 2290 cases of lung injury have been reported and 47 deaths have been confirmed with e-cigarette product use. No evidence of infectious disease has been identified. Therefore, the lung injuries are likely associated with chemical exposure; vitamin E acetate, which is used as an additive in some THC-containing vaping products, has been identified as a chemical of concern. Recent testing of bronchoalveolar lavage samples collected from patients with lung injury associated with using of vaping products identified vitamin E acetate in all samples tested; THC was found in a majority of samples.[51]

Toxic Substances – In a biomarker study in a total of 5105 subjects who provided urine samples, measurable levels of tobacco-related toxicants, including polycyclic aromatic hydrocarbons, tobacco-specific nitrosamines, and volatile organic compounds, were present in subjects who used e-cigarettes exclusively, but the levels were lower than those found in tobacco cigarette users. The highest levels of toxicants were found in dual e-cigarette and tobacco cigarette users.[42]

In a chemical analysis of e-cigarette emissions, potentially carcinogenic toxicants such as propylene oxide and glycidol were found in e-liquids and vapors; toxicant levels were highest with use of devices that reached higher temperatures (e.g., single-coil vs double-coil vaporizers) and devices that had residue buildup.[43] The vapor from e-cigarettes has also been found to contain potentially toxic and carcinogenic substances at levels lower than those found in cigarette smoke, but higher than those in ambient air.[44-46]

In 2 studies that performed bronchoscopies and collected induced sputum samples, changes in epithelial cells and defense proteins were detected more frequently in the lungs of e-cigarette users compared to nonsmokers.[47,48] In an *in vitro* study, endothelial cells exposed to e-cigarette vapors showed significantly decreased cell viability, increased levels of reactive oxygen species, and other markers of endothelial cell dysfunction.[49]

PREGNANCY — Counseling is the preferred treatment for pregnant women who smoke. Nicotine is known to cause adverse maternal and fetal effects, but NRT may be less harmful to the fetus than smoking, which has been associated with an increased incidence of low birth weight deliveries and peri- and post-natal complications. NRT can increase smoking cessation rates in late pregnancy by about 40% and, in one trial that followed infants after birth, it was associated with better developmental outcomes.[50]

Available human data on bupropion and varenicline use during pregnancy do not indicate an increased risk of major birth defects. Fetal toxicity was observed in animals given doses higher than maximum recommended human doses.

1. AL Siu et al. Behavioral and pharmacotherapy interventions for tobacco smoking cessation in adults, including pregnant women: U.S. Preventive Services Task Force Recommendation Statement. Ann Intern Med 2015; 163:622.
2. RS Barua et al. 2018 ACC expert consensus decision pathway on tobacco cessation treatment: a report of the American College of Cardiology task force on clinical expert consensus documents. J Am Coll Cardiol 2018; 72:3332.
3. J Hartmann-Boyce et al. Nicotine replacement therapy versus control for smoking cessation. Cochrane Database Syst Rev 2018; 5:CD000146.
4. AC Farley et al. Interventions for preventing weight gain after smoking cessation. Cochrane Database Syst Rev 2012; 1:CD006219.
5. N Lindson et al. Different doses, durations, and modes of delivery of nicotine replacement therapy for smoking cessation. Cochrane Database Syst Rev 2019; 4:CD013308.
6. Inhibitors and inducers of CYP enzymes and P-glycoprotein. Med Lett Drugs Ther 2017 September 18 (epub). Available at: medicalletter.org/downloads/CYP_PGP_Tables.pdf.
7. LA Kroon. Drug interactions with smoking. Am J Health Syst Pharm 2007; 64:1917.
8. GD Anderson and LN Chan. Pharmacokinetic drug interactions with tobacco, cannabinoids and smoking cessation products. Clin Pharmacokinet 2016; 55:1353.
9. JR Hughes et al. Antidepressants for smoking cessation. Cochrane Database Syst Rev 2014; 1:CD000031.

10. JT Hays and JO Ebbert. Bupropion for the treatment of tobacco dependence: guidelines for balancing risks and benefits. CNS Drugs 2003; 17:71.
11. Varenicline (Chantix) for tobacco dependence. Med Lett Drugs Ther 2006; 48:66.
12. EJ Mills et al. Comparisons of high-dose and combination nicotine replacement therapy, varenicline, and bupropion for smoking cessation: a systematic review and multiple treatment meta-analysis. Ann Med 2012; 44:588.
13. K Cahill et al. Pharmacological interventions for smoking cessation: an overview and network meta-analysis. Cochrane Database Syst Rev 2013; 5:CD009329.
14. TB Baker et al. Effects of nicotine patch vs varenicline vs combination nicotine replacement therapy on smoking cessation at 26 weeks: a randomized clinical trial. JAMA 2016; 315:371.
15. AS Gershon et al. Cardiovascular and neuropsychiatric events after varenicline use for smoking cessation. Am J Respir Crit Care Med 2018; 197:913.
16. D Kotz et al. Cardiovascular and neuropsychiatric risks of varenicline: a retrospective cohort study. Lancet Respir Med 2015; 3:761.
17. JR Hughes. Varenicline as a cause of suicidal outcomes. Nicotine Tob Res 2016; 18:2.
18. RM Anthenelli et al. Effects of varenicline on smoking cessation in adults with stably treated current or past major depression: a randomized trial. Ann Intern Med 2013; 159:390.
19. AE Evins et al. Maintenance treatment with varenicline for smoking cessation in patients with schizophrenia and bipolar disorder: a randomized clinical trial. JAMA 2014; 311:145.
20. RM Anthenelli et al. Neuropsychiatric safety and efficacy of varenicline, bupropion, and nicotine patch in smokers with and without psychiatric disorders (EAGLES): a double-blind, randomised, placebo-controlled clinical trial. Lancet 2016; 387:2507.
21. MB Steinberg et al. Triple-combination pharmacotherapy for medically ill smokers: a randomized trial. Ann Intern Med 2009; 150:447.
22. CF Koegelenberg et al. Efficacy of varenicline combined with nicotine replacement therapy vs varenicline alone for smoking cessation: a randomized clinical trial. JAMA 2014; 312:155.
23. JO Ebbert et al. Combination varenicline and bupropion SR for tobacco-dependence treatment in cigarette smokers: a randomized trial. JAMA 2014; 311:155.
24. JE Rose and FM Behm. Combination varenicline/bupropion treatment benefits highly dependent smokers in an adaptive smoking cessation paradigm. Nicotine Tob Res 2017; 19:999.
25. M Siahpush et al. Association between duration of use of pharmacotherapy and smoking cessation: findings from a national survey. BMJ Open 2015; 5:e006229.
26. RA Schnoll et al. Long-term nicotine replacement therapy: a randomized clinical trial. JAMA Intern Med 2015; 175:504.
27. N Lindson-Hawley et al. Gradual reduction vs abrupt cessation as a smoking cessation strategy in smokers who want to quit. JAMA 2013; 310:91.
28. N Lindson-Hawley et al. Reduction versus abrupt cessation in smokers who want to quit. Cochrane Database Syst Rev 2012; 11:CD008033.
29. N Lindson-Hawley et al. Gradual versus abrupt smoking cessation: a randomized, controlled noninferiority trial. Ann Intern Med 2016; 164:585.
30. JA Cunningham et al. Effect of mailing nicotine patches on tobacco cessation among adult smokers: a randomized clinical trial. JAMA Intern Med 2016; 176:184.

31. EC Donny et al. Randomized trial of reduced-nicotine standards for cigarettes. N Engl J Med 2015; 373:1340.

32. SD Halpern et al. A pragmatic trial of e-cigarettes, incentives, and drugs for smoking cessation. N Engl J Med 2018; 378:2302.

33. SD Halpern et al. Randomized trial of four financial-incentive programs for smoking cessation. N Engl J Med 2015; 372:2108.

34. C Bullen et al. Electronic cigarettes for smoking cessation: a randomised controlled trial. Lancet 2013; 382:1629.

35. P Hajek et al. A randomized trial of e-cigarettes versus nicotine-replacement therapy. N Engl J Med 2019; 380:629.

36. S Kalkhoran and SA Glantz. E-cigarettes and smoking cessation in real-world and clinical settings: a systematic review and meta-analysis. Lancet Respir Med 2016; 4:116.

37. J Hartmann-Boyce et al. Electronic cigarettes for smoking cessation. Cochrane Database Syst Rev 2016; 9:CD010216.

38. SA Glantz and DW Bareham. E-Cigarettes: use, effects on smoking, risks, and policy implications. Annu Rev Public Health 2018; 39:215.

39. T Alzahrani et al. Association between electronic cigarette use and myocardial infarction. Am J Prev Med 2018; 55:455.

40. L McCauley et al. An unexpected consequence of electronic cigarette use. Chest 2012; 141:1110.

41. JL Barrington-Trimis et al. E-cigarettes, cigarettes, and the prevalence of adolescent tobacco use. Pediatrics 2016; 138:e20153983.

42. ML Goniewicz et al. Comparison of nicotine and toxicant exposure in users of electronic cigarettes and combustible cigarettes. JAMA Netw Open 2018, 1:e185937.

43. M Sleiman et al. Emissions from electronic cigarettes: key parameters affecting the release of harmful chemicals. Environ Sci Technol 2016; 50:9644.

44. R Goel et al. Highly reactive free radicals in electronic cigarette aerosols. Chem Res Toxicol 2015; 28:1675.

45. L Kosmider et al. Carbonyl compounds in electronic cigarette vapors: effects of nicotine solvent and battery output voltage. Nicotine Tob Res 2014; 16:1319.

46. ML Goniewicz et al. Levels of selected carcinogens and toxicants in vapour from electronic cigarettes. Tob Control 2014; 23:133.

47. A Ghosh et al. Chronic e-cigarette exposure alters the human bronchial epithelial proteome. Am J Respir Crit Care Med 2018; 198:67.

48. B Reidel et al. E-cigarette use causes a unique innate immune response in the lung, involving increased neutrophilic activation and altered mucin secretion. Am J Respir Crit Care Med 2018; 197:492.

49. WH Lee et al. Modeling cardiovascular risks of e-cigarettes with human-induced pluripotent stem cell-derived endothelial cells. J Am Coll Cardiol 2019; 73:2722.

50. T Coleman et al. Pharmacological interventions for promoting smoking cessation during pregnancy. Cochrane Database Syst Rev 2015; 12:CD010078.

51. CDC. Outbreak of lung injury associated with the use of e-cigarette, or vaping, products. Available at: www.cdc.gov/tobacco/basic_information/e-cigarettes/severe-lung-disease.html. Accessed November 20, 2019.

ADVICE FOR
Travelers

Original publication date – October 2019

Patients who receive pretravel advice can reduce their risk for many travel-related conditions. Vaccines recommended for travelers are reviewed in a separate issue.[1]

TRAVELERS' DIARRHEA

Travelers' diarrhea (TD) is common in travelers to Asia, the Middle East, Africa, Mexico, and Central and South America. It is usually caused by noninvasive strains of *Escherichia coli*; infections with *Shigella* spp., *Salmonella* spp., and *Campylobacter jejuni* can also occur. Parasites and viruses are less common causes of TD, but norovirus has become more frequent in recent years.[2] Travelers to areas where hygiene is poor should wash their hands frequently and avoid consuming raw or undercooked shellfish, raw vegetables, fruit they have not peeled themselves, unpasteurized dairy products and fruit juices, cooked food not served steaming hot (dry foods such as bread are usually safe), and tap water, including ice.

TREATMENT — Mild TD – Antibiotic treatment is not recommended for patients with mild (tolerable) TD. **Loperamide** (*Imodium A-D*, and others), a synthetic opioid, is available over the counter (OTC) and by prescription as an antimotility agent; it often relieves symptoms in <24 hours, but post-treatment constipation may occur. The recommended dosage for adults is a 4-mg loading dose, then 2 mg orally after each

Advice for Travelers

Summary: Advice for Travelers

Travelers' Diarrhea (TD)

► TD is common in travelers to Asia, the Middle East, Africa, Mexico, and Central and South America.

► Loperamide (*Imodium A-D*, and others) can relieve symptoms of mild TD.

► Azithromycin (in addition to loperamide) is recommended for empiric treatment of moderate or severe TD.

► The minimally absorbed antibiotics rifamycin and rifaximin are effective for self-treatment of TD caused by noninvasive pathogens.

► Antibiotic prophylaxis of TD is generally not recommended.

Malaria

► Travelers should use protective measures against mosquito bites (e.g., insect repellents and insecticide-treated bed nets).

► Atovaquone/proguanil has been highly effective for prophylaxis of malaria, and it is well tolerated. Alternatives for prophylaxis in most areas include doxycycline, mefloquine, and tafenoquine.

► Primaquine or tafenoquine can be used to prevent relapses of *P. vivax* malaria.

► Chloroquine and mefloquine are considered safe for use during pregnancy.

Some Other Infections

► Protection against mosquito bites is the primary way to prevent infection with **dengue, Zika, and chikungunya** viruses.

► Pregnant women should avoid traveling to any area with a risk of Zika virus infection because maternal-fetal transmission can result in microcephaly and other congenital brain abnormalities.

► Travelers at increased risk of **leptospirosis** should consider prophylaxis with doxycycline.

Noninfectious Risks of Travel

► The most effective measure for preventing **acute mountain sickness (AMS)** is gradual ascent with a slow increase in sleeping elevation. Acetazolamide is recommended when rapid ascent cannot be avoided. Dexamethasone is an alternative.

► To reduce the risk of **venous thromboembolism** during long flights, travelers should exercise calf muscles and drink extra fluids. Wearing light compression stockings or receiving a single prophylactic dose of a low-molecular-weight heparin can decrease the risk of deep vein thrombosis (DVT) in high-risk travelers.

► Treatments that can decrease symptoms of **jet lag** and hasten adaptation include melatonin, the benzodiazepine receptor agonist zolpidem, the melatonin receptor agonist ramelteon, and the stimulant armodafinil.

► A transdermal patch of the antimuscarinic drug scopolamine can prevent symptoms of **motion sickness.**

loose stool (maximum of 16 mg/day). Use of much higher doses has been associated with prolongation of the QT interval, torsades de pointes, and other ventricular arrythmias. New package-size limitations and unit-dose packaging have been implemented recently by the FDA for certain OTC loperamide products to lower the risk of abuse.[3] Loperamide should not be used in children <2 years old.

Moderate or Severe TD – Antibiotic treatment is recommended for severe (incapacitating) TD, and can be considered for moderate (distressing) TD (see Table 1). Using loperamide in combination with an appropriate antibiotic can shorten the duration of illness.[4] **Azithromycin** (*Zithromax,* and generics) and **fluoroquinolones** are active against most invasive and noninvasive bacterial pathogens that cause TD. Azithromycin is now the preferred antibiotic for empiric self-treatment of moderate or severe TD.[5] A fluoroquinolone such as ciprofloxacin (*Cipro,* and others) is an alternative, but resistance to fluoroquinolones is increasing and their use has been associated with increased acquisition of multidrug-resistant pathogens such as extended-spectrum beta-lactamase-producing *Enterobacteriaceae* (ESBL-PE).[6] They should not be used for empiric treatment of TD in South and Southeast Asia where fluoroquinolone-resistant *C. jejuni* is highly prevalent.[7,8] Fluoroquinolones can also cause serious adverse effects.[9] They are not recommended for use in children or pregnant women. A single-dose regimen of azithromycin or a fluoroquinolone is preferred over a 3-day regimen for treatment of TD, but is more likely to cause nausea.[10]

The FDA has approved **rifamycin** *(Aemcolo)*, a minimally absorbed oral antibiotic, for treatment of adults with TD caused by noninvasive strains of *E. coli.*[11] It is structurally related to **rifaximin** *(Xifaxan)*, another minimally absorbed oral antibiotic that is approved for the same indication in patients ≥12 years old. Neither of these drugs should be used for treatment of TD that is complicated by fever and/or bloody stools. In a randomized, double-blind trial in adult travelers to Mexico or Guatemala with acute diarrhea, 3 days' treatment with rifamycin 388 mg twice daily shortened the duration of diarrhea by about one day compared to

Table 1. Antibiotics for Treatment of Travelers' Diarrhea[1]		
Drug[2]	Usual Adult Dosage	Cost[3]
Azithromycin[4] − generic	1 g once or divided bid[5] or 500 mg	$8.40
Zithromax (Pfizer)	once/day x 3 days	206.00
Ciprofloxacin[6,7] − generic	750 mg once[5] or 500 mg bid x 3 days	1.60
Cipro (Bayer)		34.40
Levofloxacin[4,6] − generic	500 mg once[5] or once/day x 3 days	1.20
Levaquin (Janssen)		90.10
Ofloxacin[4,6] − generic	400 mg once[5] or once/day x 3 days	49.20
Rifamycin[8] − *Aemcolo*	388 mg bid x 3 days	144.00
(Cosmo/Aries)		
Rifaximin[7] − *Xifaxan* (Salix)	200 mg tid x 3 days[9]	186.40

1. Antibiotic treatment is not recommended for patients with mild TD.
2. May be combined with loperamide (4 mg initially, followed by 2 mg after each loose stool [max 16 mg/24 hours]).
3. Approximate WAC for 3 days' treatment. WAC = wholesaler acquisition cost or manufacturer's published price to wholesalers; WAC represents a published catalogue or list price and may not represent an actual transactional price. Source: AnalySource® Monthly. September 5, 2019. Reprinted with permission by First Databank, Inc. All rights reserved. ©2019. www.fdbhealth.com/policies/drug-pricing-policy.
4. Not FDA-approved for treatment of travelers' diarrhea.
5. Single-dose treatment is preferred. If symptoms persist after 1 day, continue dosing (as recommended for 3-day regimens) for up to 3 days.
6. Resistance to fluoroquinolones is increasing and their use has been associated with increased acquisition of multidrug-resistant pathogens such as extended-spectrum beta-lactamase-producing *Enterobacteriaceae* (ESBL-PE). They can potentially cause serious adverse effects. They should not be used for empiric treatment in South and Southeast Asia where there is a high prevalence of fluoroquinolone-resistant *Campylobacter jejuni*.
7. FDA-approved for treatment of infectious diarrhea caused by enterotoxigenic *E. coli, C. jejuni, Shigella* spp., or *Salmonella typhi*.
8. Not recommended for treatment of diarrhea that is complicated by fever and/or bloody stools.
9. In a study conducted in 4 countries (Afghanistan, Djibouti, Kenya, and Honduras), a single 1650-mg dose of rifaximin (not FDA-approved) was similar in efficacy to single 500-mg doses of azithromycin or levofloxacin in patients with acute travelers' diarrhea (MS Riddle et al. Clin Infect Dis 2017; 65:2008).

placebo.[12] Both rifamycin and rifaximin appear to be similar in efficacy to ciprofloxacin for treatment of TD caused by noninvasive pathogens, with fewer adverse effects.[13,14]

Packets of **oral rehydration salts** (*Ceralyte, ORS*, and others) mixed in potable water can prevent and treat dehydration. They are available from suppliers of travel-related products and some pharmacies in the US and overseas.

PROPHYLAXIS — Travel medicine experts generally do not recommend antibiotic prophylaxis for TD because of concerns about adverse effects and development of resistance. Some travelers, however, such as persons with immunocompromising conditions, poorly controlled diabetes, or chronic renal failure, or those with time-dependent activities who cannot risk the temporary incapacitation associated with diarrhea, might benefit from prophylaxis.

In patients who require prophylaxis, **ciprofloxacin** or **levofloxacin**, given during travel (500 mg once daily for no more than 2-3 weeks) and for 2 days after return, have been effective, but current guidelines discourage their use. **Azithromycin** 250 mg once daily is a reasonable alternative. **Rifaximin** (200-1100 mg daily divided into 1-3 doses) has been shown to be effective for TD prophylaxis in clinical trials.[5] In one trial, 200 mg twice daily reduced the incidence of TD by 48% compared to placebo in travelers going to South and Southeast Asia for 6-28 days.[15] Rifamycin has not been studied for this indication.

Bismuth subsalicylate (*Pepto-Bismol*, and others), taken as 2 ounces of liquid or 2 chewable tablets (524 mg) 4 times a day for the duration of travel, can prevent diarrhea in travelers, but it is less effective than antibiotics and can cause the tongue and stools to turn black. It is not recommended for children <3 years old or for pregnant women.

INSECT BITES

To reduce the risk of infection with diseases transmitted by insect bites, travelers should use an insect repellent such as DEET on exposed skin and treat clothing (including footwear), bed nets, tents, and sleeping bags with the synthetic pyrethroid insecticide permethrin (*Duranon, Permanone*, and others).[16] Additional protective measures include wearing light-colored shirts (with long sleeves), pants and socks, and covered shoes, and sleeping in air-conditioned or screened areas.[17] Mosquitoes that transmit malaria are most active between dusk and dawn; those that transmit viruses such as dengue, Zika, and chikungunya bite during the day, particularly in the early morning and late afternoon.

MALARIA

The risk of malaria is highest in travelers to Africa, but cases have also been reported in recent years following travel to Asia, Oceania, Central and South America, the Caribbean, and the Middle East. No drug is 100% effective for prevention of malaria; travelers should use protective measures against mosquito bites in addition to prophylactic medication.[18] Travelers to malarious areas should be reminded to seek medical attention if they develop fever during their trip or within the year after their return (especially during the first 2 months). Those going to developing countries, where counterfeit and poor-quality drugs are common, should obtain antimalarial agents before travel.

ATOVAQUONE/PROGUANIL — The once-daily fixed-dose combination of atovaquone and proguanil (*Malarone*, and generics) has been highly effective for prophylaxis of malaria; treatment-related resistance has occurred, but acquisition of resistant disease by travelers appears to be rare.[19] Atovaquone/proguanil is generally the best tolerated prophylactic, but headache, GI disturbances, nightmares, insomnia, mouth ulcers, and cases of Stevens-Johnson syndrome and hepatitis have been reported.[20] Proguanil can increase the anticoagulant effect of warfarin; caution is advised when starting or stopping atovaquone/proguanil in patients taking warfarin.

CHLOROQUINE – Chloroquine, which is taken once weekly, can only be used for prophylaxis in the few areas (mainly in the Caribbean and Central America) that still have chloroquine-sensitive malaria. It can cause headache, dizziness, blurred vision, insomnia, and pruritus, and it may exacerbate psoriasis.[21]

DOXYCYCLINE – Doxycycline (*Vibramycin*, and others) is an effective once-daily alternative for malaria prophylaxis. It frequently causes GI disturbances and can cause photosensitivity, esophagitis, and vaginitis.

Table 2. Countries with a Risk of Malaria[1]

AFRICA[2]

Angola	Eritrea[3]	Nigeria
Benin	Ethiopia[3]	Rwanda
Botswana[3]	Gabon	São Tomé
Burkina Faso	Gambia, The	and Príncipe
Burundi	Ghana	Senegal
Cameroon	Guinea	Sierra Leone
Central African	Guinea-Bissau	Somalia
Republic	Kenya[3]	South Africa[3]
Chad	Liberia	South Sudan
Comoros	Madagascar[3]	Sudan
Congo, Republic of the	Malawi	Swaziland
Côte d'Ivoire	Mali	Tanzania
Democratic Republic	Mauritania	Togo
of the Congo	Mozambique	Uganda
Djibouti	Namibia	Zambia
Equatorial Guinea	Niger	Zimbabwe

AMERICAS[2]

Bolivia[3,5]	French Guiana[3]	Nicaragua[4]
Brazil[3]	Guatemala[3-5]	Panama[3-5]
Colombia[3]	Guyana[3]	Peru[3]
Dominican	Haiti[4]	Suriname
Republic[3,4]	Honduras[3-5]	Venezuela[3]
Ecuador[3]	Mexico[4,5]	

ASIA[2]

Afghanistan	Korea, North[4,5]	Philippines[3]
Bangladesh[3]	Korea, South[3-5]	Saudi Arabia[3]
Burma (Myanmar)[3,6]	Laos[3,6]	Thailand[3,5]
Cambodia[3,6]	Malaysia[3]	Timor-Leste
India	Myanmar (Burma)[3,5]	(East Timor)
Indonesia[3]	Nepal[3]	Vietnam[3,6]
Iran[3]	Pakistan	Yemen[3]

OCEANIA

Papua New Guinea	Solomon Islands	Vanuatu

1. Only includes countries for which prophylaxis is recommended. Regional variation in risk may exist within a country. Updated detailed information is available at www.cdc.gov/malaria/travelers/country_table/a.html.
2. Unless otherwise indicated, the drugs recommended for prophylaxis include atovaquone/proguanil, doxycycline, mefloquine, and tafenoquine.
3. No malaria in major urban areas.
4. Chloroquine is an option and should generally be the drug of choice for prophylaxis.
5. Primaquine is an option for prophylaxis (based on CDC recommendation; not FDA-approved for this indication).
6. Mefloquine resistance has been reported in some areas (see Table 3 footnote 11).

Doxycycline should not be taken concurrently with antacids, oral iron, or bismuth salts (including *Pepto-Bismol*). It should not be used for malaria prophylaxis in children ≤8 years old.

MEFLOQUINE – Mefloquine is effective for malaria prophylaxis, and it has the advantage of once-weekly dosing. Travelers taking mefloquine are more likely to report dizziness, insomnia, anxiety, depressed mood, and abnormal dreams than those taking other antimalarials.[22] The drug appears to be well tolerated in children, with a low incidence of CNS adverse effects.[23] Mefloquine is contraindicated in patients with a history of a psychiatric disorder (including severe anxiety and depression) or seizures. If a patient develops psychological or behavioral abnormalities while taking mefloquine, another drug should be substituted. ECG changes have been reported in patients receiving mefloquine; the drug should be used with caution in those with cardiac conduction abnormalities.

Ketoconazole, a strong inhibitor of CYP3A4, should not be taken with or within 15 weeks after mefloquine because of a risk of fatal prolongation of the QT interval. Other drugs that are strong or moderate inhibitors of CYP3A4 may also increase mefloquine serum concentrations and the risk of QT interval prolongation. Inducers of CYP3A4, such as rifampin and carbamazepine, could reduce mefloquine serum concentrations and its efficacy.[24] Use of mefloquine with related antimalarials such as quinine, quinidine, or chloroquine, or with other drugs that prolong the QT interval, is not recommended.[25]

PRIMAQUINE – Primaquine phosphate is the most effective drug for preventing *P. vivax* malaria. It is a once-daily alternative for prophylaxis in areas where *P. vivax* is the predominant species. Primaquine is some-what less effective than other drugs against *P. falciparum*, but it can be used when other prophylactic drugs are not tolerated or are contraindicated.[21] Primaquine is also used for "terminal prophylaxis" after departure from areas where *P. vivax* and *Plasmodium ovale* are endemic (see Table 3, footnote 4). Primaquine can cause hemolytic anemia in patients with glucose-6-phosphate dehydrogenase (G6PD) deficiency, which is most common in African, Asian, and Mediterranean peoples. Travelers should be screened for G6PD deficiency before taking the drug (since available tests may fail to identify some persons at risk of hemolysis, monitoring for signs of acute hemolysis, such as jaundice, pallor, and dark urine, is recommended).

TAFENOQUINE – The FDA has approved tafenoquine, a long-acting analog of primaquine, for prophylaxis of malaria in adults (*Arakoda;* 100-mg tablets), and for prevention of relapse of *P. vivax* malaria in patients ≥16 years old undergoing treatment for acute *P. vivax* infection (*Krintafel;* 150-mg tablets). Tafenoquine is active against all stages of the malaria parasite and all species of malaria. In clinical trials, once-weekly tafenoquine was generally comparable in efficacy to mefloquine for prophylaxis of *P. falciparum* malaria. A single dose of tafenoquine was generally comparable to 14 days of primaquine for prevention of recurrence of *P. vivax* parasitemia in patients with confirmed *P. vivax* infection. Like primaquine, tafenoquine is contraindicated in persons with G6PD deficiency.[26] Corneal deposits (vortex keratopathy) that did not result in vision changes and psychiatric adverse effects have been reported with use of tafenoquine for prophylaxis.[27]

CHOICE OF DRUGS FOR PROPHYLAXIS — Factors to consider in choosing an antimalarial agent for prophylaxis include drug resistance in the area of travel, length of travel, dosing regimen, adverse effects, and cost (see recommendations for specific countries in Table 2). In the few areas (mainly in the Caribbean and Central America) that still have **chloroquine-sensitive malaria**, chloroquine is generally considered the drug of choice for prophylaxis. Atovaquone/proguanil, doxycycline, mefloquine, or tafenoquine can also be used for prophylaxis in these areas and they are recommended for prophylaxis in the many areas with **chloroquine-resistant malaria.** Primaquine is an option in the few areas where *P. vivax* is the predominant species. Atovaquone/proguanil, doxycycline, and tafenoquine can be used for prophylaxis against **mefloquine-resistant malaria**, which occurs in parts of Southeast Asia. Primaquine and tafenoquine are the only drugs that can prevent *P. vivax* **relapses**, which arise from the parasite's dormant

Table 3. Drugs for Malaria Prophylaxis[1,2]

Drug	Adult Dosage
All *Plasmodium* species in chloroquine-sensitive areas[4,5]	
Chloroquine phosphate[6,7] – generic	500 mg (300 mg base) once/wk
All *Plasmodium* species in chloroquine-resistant areas[4,5]	
Atovaquone/proguanil – generic *Malarone (GSK); Malarone Pediatric*	1 adult tablet (250 mg/100 mg) once/day[8,9]
Doxycycline[12] – generic *Vibramycin (Pfizer)*	100 mg once/day

1. No drug guarantees protection against malaria. Travelers should be advised to seek medical attention if fever develops during travel or after they return. Insect repellents, insecticide-impregnated bed nets, and proper clothing are important adjuncts for malaria prophylaxis.
2. Based on CDC recommendations. Some of these drugs may not be FDA-approved for prophylaxis of the malaria species for which they are recommended.
3. Approximate WAC for a 4-week trip at the lowest usual adult dosage. WAC = wholesaler acquisition cost or manufacturer's published price to wholesalers; WAC represents a published catalogue or list price and may not represent an actual transactional price. Source: AnalySource® Monthly. September 5, 2019. Reprinted with permission by First Databank, Inc. All rights reserved. ©2019. www.fdbhealth.com/policies/drug-pricing-policy.
4. Chloroquine-resistant *P. falciparum* occurs in all malarious areas except the Caribbean and Central America west of the Panama Canal. *P. vivax* with decreased susceptibility to chloroquine has been confirmed in Papua New Guinea and Indonesia.
5. If another drug is used for primary prophylaxis, primaquine or tafenoquine can be given after departure from areas where *P. vivax* or *P. ovale* is endemic for prevention of a possible relapse after infection with these species (Presumptive Anti-Relapse Therapy [PART], "terminal prophylaxis"). The dosage of primaquine phosphate recommended by the CDC is 30 mg base once/day (0.5 mg/kg base/day for children) for 14 days (FDA-approved dosage is 15 mg/day x 14 days). One clinical trial found that a 7-day high-dose (1 mg/kg/day) course of primaquine was noninferior to a 14-day course (0.5 mg/kg/day) for prevention of recurrence of *P. vivax* malaria (WRJ Taylor et al. Lancet 2019; 394:929). A single 300-mg dose of tafenoquine (*Krintafel*) is recommended for PART by the CDC and is FDA-approved (in combination with antimalarial therapy) to prevent relapses in patients ≥16 years old undergoing treatment for acute *P. vivax* infection. See also footnote 15. Most malarious areas (except the Caribbean) have at least 1 species of relapsing malaria. PART is generally indicated only for persons who have had prolonged exposure in malaria-endemic areas (e.g., missionaries, military personnel, Peace Corps volunteers).

Pediatric Dosage	Duration	Cost[3]
5 mg/kg base (300 mg max) once/wk	Start: 1-2 wks before travel Stop: 4 wks after leaving malarious zone	$60.30
5-8 kg: ½ ped tab/day[8,10] 9-10 kg: ¾ ped tab/day[8,10] 11-20 kg: 1 ped tab/day[8] 21-30 kg: 2 ped tabs/day[8] 31-40 kg: 3 ped tabs/day[8] >40 kg: 1 adult tab/day[8]	Start: 1-2 days before travel Stop: 1 wk after leaving malarious zone[11]	194.00 242.30
≥8 yrs: 2.2 mg/kg once/day up to 100 mg/day[13]	Start: 1-2 days before travel Stop: 4 wks after leaving malarious zone	59.90 681.70

6. Alternatives for patients who are unable to take chloroquine include atovaquone/proguanil, mefloquine, doxycycline, tafenoquine or (in a few areas) primaquine (see Table 2) dosed as for chloroquine-resistant areas.
7. Chloroquine should be taken with food to decrease GI adverse effects. If chloroquine phosphate is not available, hydroxychloroquine sulfate is as effective; 400 mg of hydroxychloroquine sulfate is equivalent to 500 mg of chloroquine phosphate.
8. Atovaquone/proguanil is available as a fixed-dose combination tablet: adult tablets (*Malarone*, and generics; 250 mg atovaquone/100 mg proguanil) and pediatric tablets (*Malarone Pediatric*, and generics; 62.5 mg atovaquone/25 mg proguanil). To enhance absorption and reduce nausea and vomiting, it should be taken with food or a milky drink. The drug should not be given to patients with severe renal impairment (creatinine clearance <30 mL/min).
9. Less frequent dosing (once or twice weekly) has also been effective in preventing malaria (GA Deye et al. Clin Infect Dis 2012; 54:232;T Lachish et al. J Travel Med 2016; 23[6]).
10. Dosage recommended by the CDC. Not FDA-approved for prevention of malaria in children weighing <11 kg.
11. Some travel medicine experts now recommend stopping atovaquone/proguanil 3 days after exposure ends. The results of one study suggest that discontinuation 1 day after exposure ends is effective (E Leshem et al. J Travel Med 2014; 21:82).
12. Doxycycline should be taken with adequate water to avoid esophageal irritation. It can be taken with food to minimize GI adverse effects. It should not be used for malaria prophylaxis in children <8 years old.
13. Dosage recommended by the CDC. The FDA-approved dosage is 2 mg/kg/day.

Continued on next page

Table 3. Drugs for Malaria Prophylaxis[1,2] (continued)	
Drug	**Adult Dosage**
Mefloquine[14,15] – generic	250 mg once/wk[16]
Primaquine phosphate[19,20] – generic	30 mg base once/day
Tafenoquine[19] – *Arakoda* (Sixty Degrees)	200 mg once/wk[21]

14. Mefloquine should be used with caution in patients with conduction abnormalities. It should not be taken on an empty stomach, and should be taken with at least 8 ounces of water.
15. Mefloquine should only be used in areas with mefloquine-sensitive malaria. Resistance to mefloquine has been confirmed in parts of Southeast Asia: on the borders of Thailand with Burma (Myanmar) and Cambodia, in the western provinces of Cambodia, in the eastern states of Burma on the border between Burma and China, along the borders of Laos and Burma, the adjacent parts of the Thailand-Cambodia border, in southern Vietnam.
16. In the US, a 250-mg tablet of mefloquine contains 228 mg mefloquine base. Outside the US, each 275-mg tablet contains 250 mg base.
17. For pediatric doses <½ tablet, it is advisable to have a pharmacist crush the tablet, estimate doses by weighing, and package them in gelatin capsules. There are no data on use in children <5 kg, but based on dosages in other weight groups, a dose of 5 mg/kg can be used.

hypnozoite stage in the liver and can occur in travelers who received primary prophylaxis with atovaquone/proguanil, mefloquine, or doxycycline and did not develop symptoms of *P. vivax* malaria soon after exposure.[28]

PREGNANCY — Malaria in pregnancy is particularly serious for both mother and fetus; prophylaxis is indicated if travel cannot be avoided. **Chloroquine** has been used extensively and safely for prophylaxis of chloroquine-sensitive malaria during pregnancy. **Mefloquine** is recommended for prophylaxis of chloroquine-resistant malaria in pregnant women; it is considered safe for use during any trimester of pregnancy.[29] The safety of **atovaquone/proguanil** in pregnancy has not been established, and its use is generally not recommended; the results of small prospective studies and analyses of data from a pregnancy registry and from reports to the manufacturer on birth outcomes following accidental

Pediatric Dosage	Duration	Cost[3]
≤9 kg: 5 mg/kg salt once/wk[17] 10-19 kg: ¼ tab once/wk[17] 20-30 kg: ½ tab once/wk 31-45 kg: ¾ tab once/wk >45 kg: 1 tab once/wk	Start: ≥2 wks before travel[18] Stop: 4 wks after leaving malarious zone	$79.40
0.5 mg/kg base once/day	Start: 1-2 days before travel Stop: 1 wk after leaving malarious zone	81.20
Not approved	Start: 200 mg/day for 3 days before travel Stop: 1 wk after leaving malarious zone	285.00

18. Most adverse events occur within 3 doses. Some Medical Letter reviewers favor starting mefloquine 3-4 weeks prior to travel and monitoring the patient for adverse events; this allows time to change to an alternative regimen if mefloquine is not tolerated.
19. Patients should be screened for G6PD deficiency before starting treatment. Should be taken with food to minimize nausea and abdominal pain.
20. Not FDA-approved for prophylaxis of malaria. Recommended by the CDC for primary prophylaxis in areas with >90% P. vivax malaria.
21. Beginning 7 days after last starting dose. Continuous dosing for >6 months is not recommended.

exposure do not suggest a teratogenic effect.[30] Proguanil alone has been used in pregnancy without evidence of toxicity. Use of **doxycycline**, **primaquine**, or **tafenoquine** during pregnancy is contraindicated.

SOME OTHER INFECTIONS

DENGUE, ZIKA, AND CHIKUNGUNYA — Dengue, Zika, and chikungunya viruses are transmitted by mosquito bites. Disease caused by these viruses occurs worldwide in tropical and subtropical areas, including cities.[31-33] Prevention of mosquito bites is the primary way to protect against dengue, Zika, and chikungunya virus infection. The FDA has approved a live-attenuated dengue vaccine (*Dengvaxia* – Sanofi Pasteur); it is indicated only for use in children 9-16 years old with laboratory-confirmed previous dengue infection who live in endemic areas, and it is not expected to be available until 2020. Pregnant women should avoid traveling to any area with a risk of Zika virus infection because maternal-fetal transmission can result in microcephaly and other congenital brain abnormalities.[34]

LEPTOSPIROSIS — Leptospirosis, a bacterial disease that occurs in many domestic and wild animals, is endemic worldwide, but the highest incidence is in tropical and subtropical areas, particularly South and Southeast Asia, Oceania, the Caribbean, and parts of sub-Saharan Africa and Central and South America. Transmission to humans usually occurs through contact with fresh water or damp soil contaminated by the urine of infected animals, particularly after heavy rainfall or flooding.[35] Travelers at increased risk, such as those who engage in adventure races, caving, or recreational water activities such as whitewater rafting, should consider prophylaxis with doxycycline 200 mg once weekly, beginning 1-2 days before and continuing throughout the period of exposure.[36]

NONINFECTIOUS RISKS OF TRAVEL

Many noninfectious health risks are associated with travel. The majority of travel-related deaths are caused by traffic accidents, drowning, falls from heights, murder, and suicide.

ACUTE ALTITUDE ILLNESS — Rapid exposure to high altitudes can cause acute mountain sickness (AMS); symptoms include headache, fatigue, nausea, anorexia, sleep disturbance, and dizziness. Travelers may also develop high altitude cerebral edema (HACE), a severe form of AMS, or high altitude pulmonary edema (HAPE).

The most effective preventive measure for AMS and HACE is gradual ascent with a slow increase in sleeping elevation. Travelers to altitudes of 2500-3000 m can lower the risk of AMS by sleeping 1 night at an intermediate altitude. At altitudes >3000 m, sleeping elevation should not increase more than 300-500 m per night.[37] If rapid ascent cannot be avoided, prophylaxis should be considered.

Acetazolamide, a carbonic anhydrase inhibitor taken in a dosage of 125 mg twice daily beginning the day before ascent, decreases the incidence and severity of AMS. The drug should be continued for 2-4 days (depending on the rate of ascent) after arrival at the target altitude; those who are climbing a peak should continue treatment until they start to descend.[38] The recommended dose for children is 2.5 mg/kg (max 125 mg) every 12 hours. Although acetazolamide, a nonantibacterial sulfonamide, is not expected to cross-react with sulfonamide antibiotics, hypersensitivity reactions to acetazolamide have been documented in those who have had severe (life-threatening) allergic reactions to sulfonamide antibiotics.[39,40]

Dexamethasone (*Decadron*, and others) 2 mg every 6 hours or 4 mg every 12 hours has also been shown to prevent AMS in adults. It is not recommended for prophylaxis in children. **Ibuprofen** 600 mg every 8 hours started a few hours before ascent can prevent high-altitude head-ache.[41] In a randomized trial in adult volunteers ascending to 3810 m, ibuprofen was slightly inferior to acetazolamide for AMS prevention (AMS incidence 62.2% vs 51.1%).[42]

Pharmacologic prophylaxis of HAPE should generally only be considered for persons with a history of HAPE.[37] Extended-release **nifedipine** (*Procardia XL*, and others) 30 mg every 12 hours started the day before ascent is recommended. **Tadalafil** (*Cialis,* and others) 10 mg every 12 hours is an alternative.[43] In one study, addition of tadalafil to acetazolamide reduced the incidence of severe altitude illness, mainly HAPE, in travelers with no prior history of HAPE.[44]

VENOUS THROMBOEMBOLISM — Prolonged immobilization during travel, particularly air travel, increases the risk of lower extremity deep vein thrombosis (DVT) and pulmonary embolism. Travelers with risk factors for thrombosis (past history of thrombosis, recent surgery, severe obesity, active malignancy, pregnancy, estrogen use, advanced age, limited mobility, thrombophilic disorders, increased platelets) are at higher risk.[45] Nevertheless, flight-related symptomatic pulmonary embolism is rare.[46]

To minimize the risk, travelers taking long-distance flights (>6 hours) should be advised to procure an aisle seat, walk around frequently, exercise calf muscles while sitting, and drink extra fluids.[47] Properly fitted light compression stockings can decrease the risk of asymptomatic DVT.[48] In one trial, giving a single prophylactic dose of a low-molecular-weight heparin to travelers at high risk reduced the incidence of DVT.[49]

JET LAG — Disturbance of body and environmental rhythms resulting from rapidly crossing multiple time zones gives rise to jet lag, which is characterized by insomnia, daytime sleepiness, decreased quality of sleep, exhaustion, loss of concentration, irritability, and GI disturbances. It is usually more severe after eastward travel.[50]

Shifting daily activities to correspond to the time zone of the destination country before arrival along with taking short naps, remaining well hydrated, avoiding alcohol, and pursuing activities in sunlight on arrival may be helpful. Several treatments that can decrease symptoms and hasten adaptation are available.[51] A program of appropriately timed light exposure and avoidance in the new time zone may adjust the "body clock" and reduce jet lag. The dietary supplement **melatonin** (0.5-5 mg started 30-60 minutes before bedtime on the first night of travel and continued for 1-5 days after arrival) has been reported to facilitate the shift of the sleep-wake cycle and decrease symptoms in some patients.[52] Taking the benzodiazepine receptor agonist **zolpidem** *(Ambien, and others)* or the melatonin receptor agonist **ramelteon** *(Rozerem)* on the first night after eastward travel and continuing for 3-4 nights has helped improve sleep.[53,54] In patients with experimentally-induced jet lag, **tasimelteon** *(Hetlioz),* another melatonin receptor agonist, significantly decreased sleep latency and improved sleep efficiency and total sleep time.[55]

The stimulants **modafinil** *(Provigil)* and **armodafinil** *(Nuvigil)* can maintain alertness in jet lag. A randomized, double-blind trial found that taking armodafinil in the morning for 3 days after eastward travel through 6 time zones increased daytime wakefulness.[56]

MOTION SICKNESS — Drug therapies for motion sickness are limited. A transdermal patch of the prescription anticholinergic **scopolamine** (*Transderm Scop*, and generics) placed behind the ear 6-8 hours before exposure to a stimulus and changed, alternating ears, every 3 days can prevent symptoms, and is better tolerated than a highly sedating antihistamine such as **promethazine** (*Phenergan*, and others).[57] OTC first-generation antihistamines such as **dimenhydrinate** (*Dramamine*, and others) and **meclizine** (*Bonine*, and others) are less effective, but may be helpful for milder symptoms.[58]

SUNBURN — Use of a broad-spectrum (both UVA and UVB protective) sunscreen with a sun protection factor (SPF) of ≥15 is generally recommended for adults and children ≥6 months old during any sun exposure that might burn unprotected skin. For maximum efficacy, sunscreen should be applied about 15-30 minutes before sun exposure and reapplied at least every 2 hours and after swimming or sweating. When using both sunscreen and insect repellent, the sunscreen should be applied first.[59] Travelers should also wear sun-protective clothing such as pants, long-sleeved shirts, and hats (fabrics with tighter weaves such as denim offer the best protection) and sunglasses, and should avoid, if possible, direct sun exposure during peak hours (10 am–4 pm).

1. Vaccines for travelers. Med Lett Drugs Ther 2018; 60:185.
2. NJ Ajami et al. Seroepidemiology of norovirus-associated travelers' diarrhea. J Travel Med 2014; 21:6.
3. FDA In Brief: FDA approves new packaging for brand-name over-the-counter loperamide to help curb abuse and misuse. September 20, 2019. Accessed September 26, 2019.
4. MS Riddle et al. Effect of adjunctive loperamide in combination with antibiotics on treatment outcomes in traveler's diarrhea: a systematic review and meta-analysis. Clin Infect Dis 2008; 47:1007.
5. MS Riddle et al. Guidelines for the prevention and treatment of travelers' diarrhea: a graded expert panel report. J Travel Med 2017; 24(suppl 1):S63.
6. R Steffen et al. Traveler's diarrhea: a clinical review. JAMA 2015; 313:71.
7. D Jain et al. Campylobacter species and drug resistance in a north Indian rural community. Trans R Soc Trop Med Hyg 2005; 99:207.
8. DR Tribble et al. Traveler's diarrhea in Thailand: randomized, double-blind trial comparing single-dose and 3-day azithromycin-based regimens with a 3-day levofloxacin regimen. Clin Infect Dis 2007; 44:338.

9. In brief: More fluoroquinolone warnings. Med Lett Drugs Ther 2018; 60:136.

10. MS Riddle et al. Trial evaluating ambulatory therapy of travelers' diarrhea (TrEAT TD) study: a randomized controlled trial comparing 3 single-dose antibiotic regimens with loperamide. Clin Infect Dis 2017; 65:2008.

11. Rifamycin (Aemcolo) for treatment of travelers' diarrhea. Med Lett Drugs Ther 2019; 61:39.

12. HL DuPont et al. Targeting of rifamycin SV to the colon for treatment of travelers' diarrhea: a randomized, double-blind, placebo-controlled phase 3 study. J Travel Med 2014; 21:369.

13. KS Hong and JS Kim. Rifaximin for the treatment of acute infectious diarrhea. Therap Adv Gastroenterol 2011; 4:227.

14. R Steffen et al. Rifamycin SV-MMX for treatment of travellers' diarrhea: equally effective as ciprofloxacin and not associated with the acquisition of multi-drug resistant bacteria. J Travel Med 2018; 25(1).

15. P Zanger et al. Effectiveness of rifaximin in prevention of diarrhoea in individuals travelling to south and southeast Asia: a randomised, double-blind, placebo-controlled, phase 3 trial. Lancet Infect Dis 2013; 13:946.

16. Insect repellents. Med Lett Drugs Ther 2019; 61:129.

17. E Mirzaian et al. Mosquito-borne illnesses in travelers: a review of risk and prevention. Pharmacotherapy 2010; 30:1031.

18. DO Freedman et al. Medical considerations before international travel. N Engl J Med 2016; 375:247.

19. HM Staines et al. Clinical implications of Plasmodium resistance to atovaquone/proguanil: a systematic review and meta-analysis. J Antimicrob Chemother 2018; 73:581.

20. PJ van Genderen et al. The safety and tolerance of atovaquone/proguanil for the long-term prophylaxis of plasmodium falciparum malaria in non-immune travelers and expatriates [corrected]. J Travel Med 2007; 14:92.

21. LC Steinhardt et al. Review: malaria chemoprophylaxis for travelers to Latin America. Am J Trop Med Hyg 2011; 85:1015.

22. M Tickell-Painter et al. Mefloquine for preventing malaria during travel to endemic areas. Cochrane Database Syst Rev 2017; 10:CD006491.

23. P Schlagenhauf et al. Use of mefloquine in children – a review of dosage, pharmacokinetics and tolerability data. Malar J 2011; 10:292.

24. Inhibitors and inducers of CYP enzymes and P-glycoprotein. Med Lett Drugs Ther 2019 September 20 (epub). Available at: medicalletter.org/downloads/CYP_PGP_Tables.pdf.

25. RL Woosley et al. QT drugs list, AZCERT, Inc. Available at www.credibleMeds.org. Accessed September 26, 2019.

26. CS Chu and DO Freedman. Tafenoquine and G6Pd: a primer for clinicians. J Travel Med 2019; 26(4).

27. Tafenoquine (Arakoda; Krintafel) for malaria. Med Lett Drugs Ther 2019; 61:101.

28. E Meltzer et al. Vivax malaria chemoprophylaxis: the role of atovaquone-proguanil compared to other options. Clin Infect Dis 2018; 66:1751.

29. P Schlagenhauf et al. Pregnancy and fetal outcomes after exposure to mefloquine in the pre- and periconception period and during pregnancy. Clin Infect Dis 2012; 54:e124.

30. RC Mayer et al. Safety of atovaquone-proguanil during pregnancy. J Travel Med 2019; 26(4).
31. MG Guzman and E Harris. Dengue. Lancet 2015; 385:453.
32. MK Kindhauser et al. Zika: the origin and spread of a mosquito-borne virus. Bull World Health Organ 2016; 94:675.
33. SC Weaver and M Lecuit. Chikungunya virus and the global spread of a mosquito-borne disease. N Engl J Med 2015; 372:1231.
34. F Krauer et al. Zika virus infection as a cause of congenital brain abnormalities and Guillain-Barré syndrome: systematic review. PLoS Med 2017; 14(1):e1002203.
35. MA Mwachui et al. Environmental and behavioural determinants of leptospirosis transmission: a systematic review. PLoS Negl Trop Dis 2015; 9(9):e0003843.
36. ND Gundacker et al. Infections associated with adventure travel: a systematic review. Travel Med Infect Dis 2017; 16:3.
37. AM Luks et al. Wilderness Medical Society Practice Guidelines for the prevention and treatment of acute altitude illness: 2019 update. Wilderness Environ Med 2019 Jun 24 (epub).
38. EV Low et al. Identifying the lowest effective dose of acetazolamide for the prophylaxis of acute mountain sickness: systematic review and meta-analysis. BMJ 2012; 345:e6779.
39. TE Kelly and PH Hackett. Acetazolamide and sulfonamide allergy: a not so simple story. High Alt Med Biol 2010: 11:319.
40. Sulfonamide cross-reactivity. Med Lett Drugs Ther 2019; 61:44.
41. J Xiong et al. Efficacy of ibuprofen on prevention of high altitude headache: a systematic review and meta-analysis. PLoS One 2017; 12:e0179788.
42. P Burns et al. Altitude sickness prevention with ibuprofen relative to acetazolamide. Am J Med 2019; 132:247.
43. M Maggiorini et al. Both tadalafil and dexamethasone may reduce the incidence of high-altitude pulmonary edema: a randomized trial. Ann Intern Med 2006; 145:497.
44. E Leshem et al. Tadalafil and acetazolamide versus acetazolamide for the prevention of severe high-altitude illness. J Travel Med 2012; 19:308.
45. M Izadi et al. Do pregnant women have a higher risk for venous thromboembolism following air travel? Adv Biomed Res 2015; 4:60.
46. D Chandra et al. Meta-analysis: travel and risk for venous thromboembolism. Ann Intern Med 2009; 151:180.
47. JR Bartholomew and NS Evans. Travel-related venous thromboembolism. Vasc Med 2019; 24:93.
48. MJ Clarke et al. Compression stockings for preventing deep vein thrombosis in airline passengers. Cochrane Database Syst Rev 2016; 9:CD004002.
49. MR Cesarone et al. Venous thrombosis from air travel: the LON- FLIT3 study–prevention with aspirin vs low-molecular-weight heparin (LMWH) in high-risk subjects: a randomized trial. Angiology 2002; 53:1.
50. C Cingi et al. Jetlag related sleep problems and their management: a review. Travel Med Infect Dis 2018; 24:59.
51. J Arendt. Approaches to the pharmacological management of jet lag. Drugs 2018; 78:1419.

52. V Srinivasan et al. Jet lag, circadian rhythm sleep disturbances, and depression: the role of melatonin and its analogs. Adv Ther 2010; 27:796.

53. AO Jamieson et al. Zolpidem reduces the sleep disturbance of jet lag. Sleep Med 2001; 2:423.

54. PC Zee et al. Effects of ramelteon on insomnia symptoms induced by rapid, eastward travel. Sleep Med 2010; 11:525.

55. WP Williams 3rd et al. Comparative review of approved melatonin agonists for the treatment of circadian rhythm sleep-wake disorders. Pharmacotherapy 2016; 36:1028.

56. RP Rosenberg et al. A phase 3, double-blind, randomized, placebo-controlled study of armodafinil for excessive sleepiness associated with jet lag disorder. Mayo Clin Proc 2010; 85:630.

57. A Spinks and J Wasiak. Scopolamine (hyoscine) for preventing and treating motion sickness. Cochrane Database Syst Rev 2011; (6):CD002851.

58. A Koch et al. The neurophysiology and treatment of motion sickness. Dtsch Arztebl Int 2018; 115:687.

59. Sunscreens. Med Lett Drugs Ther 2018; 60:129.

Index

Index

Index

Index

Index

Lozenge, nicotine, **213,** 216. *See also* Nicotine replacement therapy
Lucentis. See Ranibizumab
Lumigan, 82
Lutein
   for age-related macular degeneration, 89
Luvox, 23
Lyme disease, 129
Lyrica. See Pregabalin

M

Macugen. See Pegaptanib sodium
Malaria
   and insect repellents, 129
   during travel, 228, 231, **232,** 238
Malarone. See Atovaquone/proguanil
MAO inhibitors, 12, 216
Marijuana. *See also* Cannabidiol
   for eye disorders, 86
MARINA, 90
Meclizine, 243
Mefloquine, 228, 234, 235, 238
Melatonin, 228, 242
Mephyton. See Vitamin K
Mercaptopurine, 108
Metformin
   combinations, 58-61
   for type 2 diabetes, **43,** 48, 50, 54, 69
Methazolamide, 81
Methotrexate
   drug interactions with, 102, 109, 171
   for psoriasis, 162, **166,** 168
   for psoriatic arthritis, 182, **183,** 186, 191, 193, 195
Methylprednisolone, 103, 105
Metipranolol, 82
Metoprolol
   for atrial fibrillation, 28, 35
   for chronic heart failure, 118, 121, 122, 126
Metronidazole, 23
Mevacor. See Lovastatin
Mexeza, 84
Miglitol, 50, 58, 62
Mipomersen, 157
Mitigare, 104. *See also* Colchicine

Modafinil
   for jet lag, 242
Monoamine oxidase inhibitors. *See* MAO inhibitors
Mosquito bites. *See* Insect repellents
Motion sickness, 228, **243**
Motrin. See Ibuprofen
Moxifloxacin, ophthalmic, 94
Multaq. See Dronedarone
MVASI. See Bevacizumab

N

N,N-diethyl-*m*-toluamide. *See* DEET
Nadolol, 28
Nafcillin, 23
Naphazoline, 208
Naphazoline/pheniramine, 208, 210
Naphcon-A. See Naphazoline/ pheniramine
Naprosyn. See Naproxen
Naproxen
   for gout, 101, 102, 104
Nardil, 12
Nasacort. See Triamcinolone acetonide, intranasal
Nasal saline, 205, 208
Nasalcrom. See Cromolyn sodium
Nateglinide, 50, 58, 62
Natrapel, 132
Neomycin, 93, 96
Neoral. See Cyclosporine
Nesina. See Alogliptin
Netarsudil, 80, 84, **85**
Netarsudil/latanoprost, 84
Neti pot, 205
Neurontin, 14
Nexavar, 23
Niacin
   for lipid lowering, 152, **154**
Niacor. See Niacin
Niaspan. See Niacin
Nicardipine, 34
NicoDerm, 216. *See also* Nicotine replacement therapy
Nicorette, 216. *See also* Nicotine replacement therapy

Index

Index

Index